GOOD SHRINK/BAD SHRINK

GOOD SHRINK/ BAD SHRINK

Richard P. Kluft

KARNAC

First published in 2014 by
Karnac Books Ltd
118 Finchley Road
London NW3 5HT

British Library Cataloguing in Publication Data

A C.I.P. for this book is available from the British Library

ISBN-13: 978-1-78220-175-5

Typeset by V Publishing Solutions Pvt Ltd., Chennai, India

www.karnacbooks.com

To my wife
Estelle Sacknoff Kluft

And to the memory of my parents
Peppy Pearl Rabiner Kluft
Jack Murry Kluft, M.D.

And to the MIAs of all nations and wars,
and those who keep their memories alive

Primum non nocere—Firstly, do no harm

—The Oath of Hippocrates of Kos
(circa 460 BCE—circa 370 BCE)

The American Psychiatric Association supports the use of psychiatric knowledge, practice and institutions only for purposes consistent with ethical evaluation and treatment, research, consultation, and education. Abuse and misuse of psychiatry occur when psychiatric knowledge, assessment, or practice is used to further illegitimate organizational, social, or political objectives.

—*American Journal of Psychiatry, 151*: 1399 (1994).
Incorporated into the American Psychiatric
Association's *Position Statement on Identification of Abuse and Misuse of Psychiatry*,
approved December, 1998

ONE

The tape continued:

So, when I went back … I mean, I promised not to, but I just had to know … I walked into my old high school in Somerset. I looked at all the trophies in the hall … I saw the picture of our state championship football team, the one I was on … Not that I was a star, or anything. Second string running back, a few series a game, like that … I wasn't there. OK, so maybe I was out that day, when they took the pictures. But the team picture was a big deal. Wouldn't I remember missing it?

As long as I was there, at the school, I mean, I figured I'd say hello to Coach Mack … A great guy. Well, someone else was in the coach's office, a big solid guy, looked like he could still play. I asked about Coach MacDonald … You know, what he was doing these days? He got an odd look on his face. "We never had a Coach MacDonald here, son," he said. Things got blurry … Then a real bad headache …

Next thing I remember, my left arm felt cold. An IV line was running into me. They said I must have had a stroke or a seizure, or an ophthalmic migraine. I don't know about that last thing.

A female voice, calm and professional, began:

> *The last one includes elements of both. It's an irregular brain event. Some blood vessels spasm and enough blood doesn't get through to some places in the brain for normal function to continue, so they start to shut down … That's ischemia. If that persists, a stroke can occur.*

A slender young woman leaned forward. Her delicate hand and wrist, adorned with drop-dead rings and an eye-catching tennis bracelet, reached out to stop the tape. Taking a deep breath, she turned to a casually dressed man slouched in his chair. For the moment, his face and expression were obscured behind the hand rubbing his forehead.

"What do you think?" she asked.

"About what?"

"What do you mean, about what?" Eve Gilchrist bit her lip. *Control yourself! Don't let him get to you!*

Eve did not want to sit in this office with this man. Following her supervisor's recommendations, she had forced herself to walk into his office with her best smile, a recording of Joe Morgan's first session clenched tightly in hand. Ten minutes in, she was fighting to keep her composure. *Let me out of this room!*

Eve risked a glance at her gold Rolex. *Move faster!* Eve urged the timepiece forward, as if it were a sluggish racehorse her silent fervor could whip into running faster, ever faster, in the home stretch.

Eve did not like Ben Jordan, director of residency training at the U's Department of Psychiatry. She avoided him whenever possible.

Two days previously, Eve had presented her tape to her supervisor, the exceedingly more affable Dr. Kane. As the tape went on, Kane grew disconcerted. He rose and walked to his window, a thoughtful expression on his face. And then

Jeffrey Kane, her kind of person, the right kind of person, handsome and impeccably dressed, smiled the smile he smiled when he wanted to look particularly kind and wise, carefully straightened his extravagantly expensive Italian tie, and instructed Eve to consult with Ben Jordan, the man she now was enduring against her will.

Jeffrey Kane was chairman of the U's Department of Psychiatry. Eve, already an adroit departmental politician, aspired to become chief resident just down the road. So, "Great idea!" she'd enthused, hoping her best smile disguised her clenched jaw and grinding molars.

"The diagnosis?"

"That can wait."

"But …"

Ben Jordan sighed. Eve Gilchrist was beautiful, elegant, slender, rich, confident, bejeweled, and overdressed. He suspected she was more style than substance. She probably had guessed his opinion. She might even know that he opposed her acceptance to the residency. Jeff Kane had overruled him.

Eve wasn't Ben Jordan's kind of person, and he wasn't hers. The daughter of a prominent diplomat, Eve always tried to offer the perfect and politically correct answer to everything. Ben found her maddening.

Ben Jordan lacked the kinds of refinement and polish Eve was raised to consider virtues. Though bright and gifted, Eve often traded on her looks and panache. Ben was a khakis and blue blazer guy who wore inelegant bright ties (*Liberty of London, for gosh sakes!*). Inexplicably, Ben's wife Elani was a glamorous fashion icon. Eve's neck and shoulders tightened. *I cannot make an impact on this man! What on earth will he say?*

"Eve, I'm less worried about his diagnosis than whether he'll come back for another session."

"What do you mean?"

"This man is bleeding in front of you. He's telling you he's beginning to feel everything he thought he knew about himself is a lie. He's confused. He's desperate to find someone who'll help him find his way out of this hellish chaos. For this man, the kind of identity you and I count on as our touchstones, the foundations of our existence, our sense of ourselves as persons ... It's fallen apart. If we see identity and self-image as mirrors, our mirrors reflect back to us a pretty good picture of who we are. But when Joe looks into his mirror, metaphorically speaking, his image is shattered. Beyond shattered—its shards are being tossed around by his turmoil—like a kaleidoscope gone crazy in a hurricane."

"And ..."

"And his problems appear to scare you. Everything you're saying to him pushes toward the organic options that were already ruled out. He asks you to help him find out who he is, and why things are the way they are. You respond by trying to tell him what he is, and what he may have. I'm hearing two ships passing in the night. You're talking brain. He's talking mind."

"Dr. Jordan. I disagree. With all due respect ..."

"Dr. Gilchrist! You don't have to agree with me. Respect is optional. But you do have to give thoughtful consideration to what I'm saying before you reject it. I'm not in charge. If Dr. Kane, your supervisor, says you should do something, you're supposed to do it. If I say something, I speak as your consultant. You can take it or leave it. But you should think through my perspectives before you dismiss them and move on."

"My other supervisors have never criticized my work!"

"When I was a resident, it was assumed that everyone had something to learn. I caught my fair share of criticism along the way. Some was constructive, and some just plain nasty.

"Stick to reality, Dr. Gilchrist. Have you ever seen a case like this before?"

"No."

"Do you know what's going on and how to proceed?"

"No."

"Than it's rather unlikely that your efforts are already beyond improvement. Can we proceed?"

Eve blushed and dug her nails into her palms, hoping to hide the rage lurking under her shame. She'd never given anyone the finger—but giving Jordan the finger and storming out the door was tempting. Reason prevailed. The only route to becoming chief resident required Ben Jordan's approval. He could veto any candidate, and winning that honor meant a year of working closely with this impossible man. *Mend the fence, Eve!* she told herself, *Mend it quickly! In embassies all over the world you've smiled through horrid encounters with awful people, even brutal dictators!* Reining in her emotions, Eve reminded herself, *Stick to the game plan!*

Eve offered the best smile she could, and turned on the tape.

> *They observed me for a few hours, told me that they couldn't find anything wrong, and discharged me. It was too late to get back to Philly that evening. I figured maybe I could crash with one of my old friends. You know, from the team. All our families were close. It would be cool … I started knocking on doors, you know, where guys used to live. Nothing was right. Nobody lived where they should. People looked at me like I was crazy.*
>
> *After the third house I just started to cry. Nothing made sense. They said they'd call the cops. So I got back into my car, and drove all night back here. My roommate Marty was really worried. The next day, soon as I could get myself together, I went to Student Health. They assigned me to you.*
>
> *Well, with so many problems with your memory and your cognition, I think we will have to start with a comprehensive evaluation for problems of an organic nature …*
>
> *Didn't you hear me? I had all that done last fall.*

Well, here at University we like to repeat tests with our own personnel. They tend to be more expert, more experienced …

I'm from Massachusetts. Those tests were done at a Harvard teaching hospital in Boston, Beth Israel. I saw Dr. Chada …, Chada-something. Some long Indian name. He's a Harvard professor. I don't think folks here are going to do any better. I think I've gone crazy. (After five seconds of silence, the patient's sobs became audible.)

Eve turned off the tape. She bit her lip for a moment. For the first time, she looked Ben directly in the eyes. Her words came slowly and painfully, as if uttered against her will.

"I think I may have been wrong."

"Damn! Maybe there's a reasonable person hiding in there."

"Well …" Eve bit her tongue. *Don't blow it!* she begged herself.

"Like you said, 'Stick to reality.' How did I fool myself?"

Ben reached for a yellow Levenger pad. "I stopped taking notes a while back. Do you know why? Scratch that … Do you have any ideas, thoughts, notions?"

"No, and I'm afraid to guess."

"More character! Who'd 'a thunk it?" Ben met Eve's blush with a warm smile. "Over at Penn Lester Luborsky is doing close analyses of psychotherapy sessions, word by word, interaction by interaction. I trained there, and I'm still part of his research team. If you get about ten relational episodes from what someone says, no matter who they are talking about, and count up their components, the most common entries for each of the components form a CCRT, a Core Conflictual Relationship Theme. It generally shows the patient's prevailing dynamic. You need about ten."

"So you took notes on ten incidents from that tape?"

"Yes."

"And what is my patient saying?"

"Actually, I was studying you and what you were saying."

"Shi … I mean … No, I meant that. Shit!'"

"Well said! Learn the method, and pull it on someone yourself. But for now, here's how it breaks down. There is a person, who has a wish regarding someone or something. External and internal factors either get in the way of its being fulfilled or help to fulfill it."

"So?"

"For you, it might be, 'I want others to see me as poised and in control so I bypass upsetting feelings in myself and others.'"

"What's wrong with that?"

"Nothing … and everything."

"What do you mean?"

"To the extent that it's a conscious choice about how you lead your life, in a manner that keeps you distanced from true or upsetting feelings, it's fine. To the extent that you're in training to be a psychiatrist, and you need to become empathically attuned to your patients in order to understand and help them, it's an unmitigated disaster."

"But …"

"So, let me take a guess. You don't have to tell me whether I am right or wrong."

Eve wiped away a single tear. "Permission to hate your guts for all eternity?"

"Granted. You're in a psychiatry residency but you hate feelings. Or maybe you just fear them, maybe just in males. You didn't come here to be an analyst and explore the unconscious."

"No! Not at all. No!"

"Perhaps to have an exclusive and affluent practice doing psychopharm? You'd be bored silly … So I think the message is that someone very close to you often was emotionally out of control. You're trying to understand and help that kind of person. Given what little I know of your family, I doubt psychosis or heavy drugs. I would suspect that you're an ACOA gal, an adult child of alcoholics, and you'll go for a fellowship in addiction medicine. Control of feelings is big down that pathway."

Eve leaned forward and stared at Ben, "Who told you? Dr. Kane?"

Ben matched her, leaning closer and meeting her eyes. "You did. Granted, you didn't say so in so many words."

"I don't know how you figured that out," Eve sighed. "Dad is one of those drunks who's never missed a day's work, and Mom is happily sloshed most of the time. When Dad comes home and Mom greets him with a pitcher of martinis, it remains unsaid that both of them were hitting the bottle all day. Yeah, there were bad moments. Dad could get … irascible. Yes, now I wonder if I went into training to save them. Jeff picked up on that. When he confronted me, I was shocked. I guess somewhere I knew it, but I never let myself face it."

Eve wiped away more tears. "My make-up is ruined. OK. You've convinced me that Kane was right when he told me to consult you. I can see why I never wanted to work with you. Sitting here is like being forced to walk the plank and plunge into everything I run from. You keep throwing me into the deep end of the shame pool. You're dangerous."

"Well, my job is to make you dangerous, too. But let's talk about your patient. Was the rest of the session more of the same?"

"Yes. What makes people say such things?"

"Well, we've talked about why you say such things, so let's try your patient. Forget textbooks. Where would you expect to encounter the kind of things he says?"

"Really? OK. I guess in those lousy movies my ex-boyfriend dragged me to. Thrillers. Sci-fi. James Bond stuff. Nothing real."

"You know, reality and fiction have a pretty complicated relationship. Art imitates life, but life can imitate art. When the James Bond movies began coming out, some British operatives suspected movie staffers had been briefed on gimmicks they hadn't been issued yet, and actually asked why they didn't get the cool stuff Q gave James Bond."

"But what you're talking about ... You mean like the Red Chinese in *The Manchurian Candidate*?"

"No. I mean like all the 'good guy' nations that covered up their similar programs and screamed bloody murder—as if the Red Chinese were the only ones on the planet who'd do such evil things. The Red Chinese were no slouches, but they weren't first, and they had company."

"I don't believe you. Not in 1985! Not Americans! No way!"

Ben pulled an old paperback off his bookshelves. "Estabrooks's *Hypnosis*. Told tales out of school. About using hypnosis to create covert operatives who wouldn't crack under interrogation because they wouldn't know anything about their missions on a conscious level. Not too many folks took his accounts that seriously. Meanwhile, others were involved in that research up to their eyeballs, and continued the work."

"That really upsets me!"

"Good. Dr. Gilchrist, we're out of time. You might want to call that patient and tell him that you want to do a more thorough evaluation. Tell him you want to do a longer interview, a double session. Tell him that in that single session you didn't have the chance to do the kind of in-depth interview he really deserves. Say you wouldn't be surprised if he left thinking that you weren't really interested in what he was trying to tell you, and you regret that."

"And do what?"

"Try to walk in his moccasins a few minutes at a time. Don't do a swan dive into his pain, but do get close enough to learn who he is and what it's like to be him … And then you can begin to know who you are when you sit with him."

"And I was starting to like you …" Eve left wearing a genuine smile, shaking her head in disbelief. Closing the door behind her, she was surprised by the urge to dodge back in and stick her tongue out at Ben. *But that would be childish, audacious, and … Oh my God! Pretty darn flirtatious! Where did that come from? Could I like this monster? Impossible!*

Ben Jordan sat quietly. He was one of those crazy, driven teachers who savor the moments when they witness young minds taking incredible leaps into new levels of knowing. *Eve Gilchrist,* he mused, *the Plastic Barbie Doll Girl herself, opening her eyes! Who'd 'a thunk it?*

Ben sat motionless until his elation began to fade. Career teachers know they never can be sure when they'll experience this wonderful pleasure again. Finally, he chuckled, locked his files, and headed home, still smiling. A bittersweet sadness swept over him. His mother, a dedicated teacher, would have understood. A tear or two made its way down his cheek, in strange but perfect harmony with his grin.

TWO

The telephone rang four times and fell silent. A minute later it began to ring again. He answered immediately after the fourth ring.

"Hey Nick! Wanna hit Kelly's for a brew?"

"Not tonight, Marty. I have a headache."

"Turning into some frigid housewife? Well, hitting the books can give anybody a headache. Another time."

Nick barely stopped himself from throwing his phone against the wall. His eyes grew heavy. The memory of Marty's call faded quickly. He would not recall their conversation in the morning.

He tried to study, but the printed words in his text kept going out of focus. Finally, he closed his eyes and slept.

THREE

The Department of Psychiatry's monthly faculty meeting plowed through its uninspiring agenda. Box lunches as exciting as the agenda were provided. Most remained untouched and forlorn.

Jeffrey Kane sat at the head of a long conference table. His secretary, Sheila Conlan, sat to his right. Professors, associate professors, assistant professors, and instructors occupied the chairs around the long table and most of the single rows of seats behind the table seats on both sides. A cluster of folding chairs beyond the far end of the table was the traditional domain of fellows taking advanced specialized training and the more senior residents. Junior residents like Eve Gilchrist were usually too busy with clinical duties to attend.

The well-being and concerns of the faculty members fell to Jeff and his unofficial cabinet of advisors. Ben sat near Jeff. He ran the show when issues related to the residency or to the residents arose. Rarely the Curriculum Committee, a stodgy group that rotated its chairmanship in such an arcane and impenetrable manner that nobody knew who was on first, brought matters to the faculty's attention.

Sheila made several administrative announcements on Jeff's behalf. Next Len Liebowitz and Lisa Hart reported recent improvements in the psych curriculum for medical students.

Bobby Gray followed, making his first report as chief resident. The chief resident, an outstanding trainee given special responsibilities and duties under the joint supervision of Ben and Jeff, brought residents' concerns to the faculty and vice versa. Selection as chief resident was the medical equivalent of being elected "Most Likely to Succeed," the royal road to faculty appointment. Eve was already campaigning for the honor.

Bobby Gray was a kind, self-effacing wunderkind whose talent and energy appeared limitless. He hailed from rural Kentucky. Bobby's predecessor had written an essay that won him both a prize and a coveted overseas elective at London's Hampstead Clinic. He'd left for England as soon as he could.

Identifying and recruiting outside speakers for presentations in the department's Grand Rounds program was a task shared by the chief resident and an advisory committee. The chief did the real work. Most chiefs couldn't complete the roster by their late June graduations and bequeathed their loose ends and empty slots to their successors.

Bobby's predecessor's abrupt departure left Grand Rounds in limbo. He began his new duties three months early, shouldering the Grand Rounds burden in addition to his already heavy obligations. Bobby completed the entire task in three weeks. As he reviewed the roster of upcoming speakers, even the most curmudgeonly professors broke out in smiles of astonishment, surprise, and delight.

Liebowitz began to clap. The whole faculty followed. Bobby went red.

"Bobby," Jeff chuckled, "that line-up is so good that I might actually come to one or two of them.

"Well done! I don't know how you talked these folks into coming for the pittance we pay. How about you stay back a few years and persuade more luminaries to grace our hallowed halls?"

Ben followed. "Way to go, Bobby! Moving on—the distressed individual called to our attention has been counseled, and has begun appropriate therapy with a colleague we all respect and would trust to treat a family member. End of story."

"Relevant risk factors were considered and assessed?" asked Jeff.

"Absolutely."

"May I comment?" asked Bobby.

"Sure," Jeff responded.

"The residents have asked me to thank Dr. Jordan for his tactful handling of the situation."

Ben nodded to the smiles and "thumbs ups" sent his way.

"How is the Residents' Clinic doing, Ben?" Len Liebowitz asked.

"Well, Len ... That's a good question. So far, so good. But you just gave me a chance to make a pitch. This may concern the Curriculum Committee."

There were audible groans.

"Brace yourselves. Increasingly, folks are seeking out more here and now technique-oriented approaches. It might be wise to bring them into the curriculum earlier than we've been doing. Plus, we'll need to provide enough supervision so these competencies will be firmly established by their graduation. We want them to leave with a skill set that's first rate both in classic and more modern methods."

The U's orientation was primarily psychodynamic, begrudging every concession forced by the cognitive-behavioral revolution. Ben's remarks awakened even the most disinterested from their torpor.

Stuart Weisel raised his hand. Ben could count on Weisel's inevitable negativism. He cautioned himself against making that slight but seductive error in pronunciation that would call Weisel the weasel he often seemed to be.

"Ben. No resident has presented a case to me that required anything out of the ordinary." He appealed to the others. "How many of you have had cases presented to you that needed anything besides good basic therapy and meds?"

A handful of people stirred in their seats. One lonely hand was raised. It belonged to Ray Hawkes, a man so marginalized that he was often called "the Leper" behind his back. He was the only professor sitting in the distant folding chairs.

"Tony Abruzzi teaches those methods," said Jeff, "but he can't supervise all of the residents. Ben picks up the hypnosis piece. For years, Ben's been trying to convince us to move in this direction."

"Not necessary," Weisel insisted.

Ray Hawkes didn't wait to be unrecognized.

"We really need more depth in those areas."

"Waste of time," said Weisel, shaking his head.

Murmurs and vigorous nods favored Weisel's stance.

"Feeling alone on this one, Ray?" asked Jeff. "Well, I think you're right."

Suddenly everyone was alert and attentive. For half a dozen years or more only Ben Jordan had backed anything Ray proposed. Ben admired Jeff's political wiles, but he worried for Ray. Adroitly, Jeff had positioned the Leper to be thrown under the bus, should a martyr prove necessary. More privileged core faculty members, like Ben himself, now could be buffered from the unpopular ideas.

"I've been thinking along these lines myself. One of our more talented residents just picked up a puzzling case, a person who's beginning to realize that the life this person thought this person had lived is falling apart. This person may have a very unusual kind of amnesia with a false autobiographic memory. I couldn't find an absolute parallel or precedent in the books, but Ben thinks it may be like the breakdown of a secondary personality in the kind of fugue we thought pretty much died out in the nineteenth century.

Some old cases seem something like this. Ben gave me a copy of Ellenberger's *The Discovery of the Unconscious*. Great reading!"

"This person … This person …" Will Rivers chuckled. "Jeff, does this person have an age, a gender?"

Ben broke in. "Jeff just gave us a great model for stating a problem without compromising confidentiality. It ain't broke, Will. Why fix it?" *Why the hell,* Ben wondered, *is the director of a research lab sticking his nose into this? Will hasn't shown interest in any clinical issue since I've been here.*

Jeff looked around, assessing reactions.

"Back to Ray's points."

Ray understood Jeff's finesse and winced. *Whose words are going to be put in my mouth? I can't speak up without shooting myself in the foot.*

"From time to time we may need the methods Ray alludes to. The resident on the case is pretty sharp, might even become our chief resident if we let Dr. Gray graduate. Treating this case may require methods that I must say I don't know and can't teach. I'm taking myself back to school 'cause I can't lean on all of you to do what I can't do myself.

"We fulfill the American Psychiatric Association's basic requirements for a good curriculum, but we aren't teaching our residents how to take this stuff to the next level."

A calm voice with an aristocratic British accent came from the second row of chairs, midway down the table.

"But surely we can't teach our residents to handle cases that are beyond the level of anyone but an expert's expert?"

Trevor Martin was brilliant and unfailingly reasonable, so perceptive that his dissent could make Ben doubt himself. Trevor was an invaluable asset as an ally, a formidable opponent as an adversary.

"Right you are, Trevor. Bottom line. I'm going to ask the Curriculum Committee to schedule a meeting to study some options ... Who's chair right now? [*Silence was followed by cackling laughter.*] Well, you guys figure it out and let me know tomorrow. We darn well are going to fix this problem."

"And would you care to specify more precisely what that problem is?" Trevor persisted.

Will raised his hand. "I still am concerned that we're going off on a wild goose chase. We should be able to hear more about the patient at the center of this storm."

Jeff rose to the challenge. "It's a general issue. We need to train our residents well enough in every modality so that beyond knowing the bare bones basics, they can anticipate and plan the next step, whether or not they can execute that next step themselves. That means more sophisticated teaching and supervision."

"I don't see where we fall short, Jeff." Porcine Lou Meadowcroft preferred group, marital, and family work to individual therapies. Ben considered Lou clever, but passive aggressive enough to drive him crazy.

"Well, let's do a little assessment of educational needs." Jeff pushed on. "Show of hands, please? How many of you are trained in hypnosis?"

A scattering of hands rose.

"How many of you have used it in the last say, three years?"

Only three raised their hands—Ben, Ray, and Len Liebowitz. Len gave his two "partners in crime" a humorous smirk. Ironically, all three were analysts. Psychoanalysts and hypnosis specialists generally buy into unproductive stereotypes of one another. Few mental health professionals master both.

"Of you three, how many of you could help a resident build on basics and get really sophisticated?"

All three raised their hands.

"Cognitive therapy? Beck's stuff?"

The first three were joined by another trio. Recent hires Lisa Hart and Bev Dresher were no surprise, but eyebrows were raised when the Weasel was number three. Ben gave Stuart a look of abject incredulity. Liebowitz wagged a finger in his direction. Not missing a beat, Stuart shrugged his shoulders with a self-depreciating grin. Dealing with the Weasel was complicated by his puzzling moments of normal, even likable human behavior.

"Ladies and gentlemen! We need to fix this. In addition to our capable if nebulous Curriculum Committee, whoever they are this week, we need a task force."

A number of hands shot up. Ben could anticipate the game plan of every eager volunteer. Jeff acknowledged each with a nod and paused, seemingly lost in thought.

Ben knew his chief. *The fix is in. He already has a plan!*

"Helen?" Jeff turned to Helen Bidwell, an older woman with the posture of a model, still striking and exquisitely groomed. She had not volunteered.

"Yes, Jeff?"

"Helen, you would be the perfect person to lead this task force."

"Of course, Jeff. That sounds like fun."

Ben loved to watch Jeff thread the needle just so. Helen Bidwell's clinical skills and intimidating intellect commanded international respect. Only the Leper disliked her. He refused to explain his surprising opinion to Ben.

Helen's specialty was family therapy. She often collaborated with Lou Meadowcroft. Years spent containing embattled spouses, squabbling parents, and rambunctious children was ideal preparation for her new assignment. Helen's appointment put a shot across the bow of those hoping to impose their wills on the task force. No one got by Helen, who would be sure to involve some of the new women on the faculty. Lisa and Bev may have ground their teeth in silence during the meeting, but Helen would ensure that their thoughtful voices would be heard where it counted.

As the faculty made their exits, Lisa Hart kidded Jeff affectionately, "That was one heck of a meeting." Jeff beamed. He devoured admiration. The beleaguered and usually speechless Tony Abbruzzi seemed overcome. He managed to choke out a hoarse "Thank you!" before he flushed and scooted off.

"Our behavior therapy professor needs some of his own assertiveness training. Maybe Lisa should treat him," Jeff whispered. "You know, Ben, thinking about Eve's patient may have pushed me more toward constructive change in our curriculum than all your arguments."

"Well, Jeff, it's a timely change. You may want to take some notes on the process and write it up for *Psychiatric Education*."

"Let's make it work first."

Jeff at his best, Ben reflected. *Jeff at his best*.

FOUR

Whenever Jeff mentioned Eve Gilchrist, he described her in glowing terms. Ergo, Will reasoned, if Jeff spoke highly of any resident other than Bobby Gray, it might be Eve. Will and his people had little contact with the residents. The chief resident responded to medical and psychiatric emergencies involving research subjects, so Will's team knew Bobby Gray. They nicknamed him "the Golden Boy."

Eve Gilchrist received a different kind of attention. Drawing upon the language of physics, the researchers nicknamed Eve "the Universal Attractor." All things considered, Will figured the mystery patient probably belonged to the Universal Attractor. He asked Sheila for directions to the labyrinthine maze of smallish rooms that was the Residents' Clinic. He never had been there before.

He saw Ray Hawkes's name on a door there. *Serves the fucker right, stuck in a glorified broom closet like a junior resident!* To Will Rivers, Ray was an impossibly rigid straight arrow, one of those offensively naïve Dudley Do-Rights who was always a pain in someone's ass, and one day might bring discomfort to his own.

Will found Eve in a tiny library provided for the residents, their hangout in free moments. Curled up in a beanbag chair, she was immersed in Luborsky's *Principles of Psychoanalytic Psychotherapy*.

Outwit me once, shame on you, Ben Jordan! Outwit me twice, shame on me! New Jersey born and bred Ben Jordan probably would use the "F-word," but Eve refused to sink to that level of vulgarity, even in the privacy of her own mind. She vowed to master the basic CCRT approach before she met again with either Jeff or Ben.

Completely absorbed, she tuned out the high-decibel rantings of two of her peers arguing about what Otto Kernberg was really saying in a recent paper.

"Eve, I'm Will Rivers."

Eve jumped to her feet, her book crashing to the floor. Will knelt and retrieved it for her.

"Thanks. I'm sorry. I just get so lost in what I read. You startled me."

"With all this racket going on?" He turned to the two suddenly speechless young men.

"At ease, guys. I don't understand Kernberg either."

The other residents laughed, relaxed, and resumed their conversation at a lower volume.

"Let me start again," said Will. "I'm Will Rivers."

"I know. You teach courses on methodology and statistics in the Psychology Department. I read some of your research papers in college. We don't see too much of you."

"True, true. Being in research I generally consort with geeks and trolls deep beneath the earth. But I emerge from my cave to attend departmental meetings as the token research psychologist."

They shared a laugh.

"Earlier today I heard something about a patient with memory problems. We study how the mind processes and retains information. Can I ask you about your patient?"

Eve tried to size up the situation, stifling the urge to ask Will how and what he knew about her patient. Will was not directly involved in her training, but he was a powerful player reputed to have a dangerous temper. *This is one man I can't risk antagonizing!*

"I'm sure you have a lot to offer, Dr. Rivers. You know Jeff and Ben are very firm about boundaries. I have to follow their leads."

"Rightly so."

"Without their say-so, I can't discuss the situation. I'm sure you understand."

"Of course, Eve. I would say the same thing. Or at least I would if I had my wits about me that day."

Eve smiled and relaxed. Will thought, *Damn, I'm good! That's the first big step toward getting around this girl! So focused on her book that she didn't notice me at all? High absorption correlates with high hypnotizability. That could prove useful.*

"Your caution speaks well of you. But I'm not asking for clinical information. You see, Eve, if the clinical faculty guys ask me to do something, of course I'll do it.

"But my grants stipulate that one hundred percent of my time belongs to research. If I work on anything else, I need to pay it back. I know that's complicated. In fact, on close examination, it's bizarre. But we all have rules we have to respect and live by. All I need to know is this—does this person have coverage? If not, I'll do some juggling."

"No problem, Dr. Rivers. Student insurance plus some disability coverage."

"Well, this stuff usually isn't covered by disability."

"No worries, sir. Not the usual kind of disability."

"Thanks, Eve. I'm sure you appreciate that I'm cautious when I fear getting trapped between my two masters."

"I don't see a problem."

Will's guile engaged Eve's well-practiced politeness and short-circuited her intellect. His fast-talking was calculated to distract Eve from looking too carefully at his rationales, falsehoods wrapped in the cloak of plausibility. In fact, Will had substantial time commitments teaching graduate seminars in psychology and Eve knew this, but Will had misdirected her from her own knowledge. Like most pure researchers, Will was unlicensed. He could not bill insurers for his services.

FIVE

Will struggled to make sense of several potentially disconcerting bits of information. Would they cohere into a meaningful pattern that demanded attention, or could they be disregarded? Jeff set extraordinarily high standards for protecting patient confidentiality. While that was praiseworthy, it frustrated Will's first attempts to work out whether or not he was facing a firestorm.

Probably it's nothing, but better safe than sorry! If Glenville-Rodgers's strategists later concluded Will had missed the boat and let matters slide ... *Better an ounce of prevention ... I ran Gilchrist around in circles this time, but if she* figures *out I played her, I won't be so lucky again. Unless I can tap her suggestibility.*

Will deduced from Jeff's and Eve's guarded admissions that a male student at the U was reporting massive amnesia. His picture of the life he'd thought to be his own was falling apart. He might be someone with a serious medical problem, or a veteran with service-connected disability. When he contemplated the latter possibility, Will's heart began to pound in his chest.

SIX

Will dialed a number at the Glenville-Rogers Foundation. A man he knew as Michael Johnson answered after four rings.

"Hey, Mike! I just wanted to give you a heads up about our friend Nick, Nick G."

"Gosh! I haven't heard from him in quite a while."

"He hasn't been feeling well lately. I bumped into a mutual friend. Nick just had a whole series of tests. Something about sentinel nodes being detected. That doesn't sound good."

"Shit! You never can tell in this fucking world."

"Sorry to be the bearer of bad news."

"Not your fault, Buddy! I'll give Nick a call."

The Program never used codes that were obviously codes. What need would a patriotic think-tank have for covert and cryptic communications?

Under Johnson, Will oversaw three operatives, codenames Nick C., Nick G., and Nick W. The Program's Nick G. was Joe Morgan, a student at the U. Was Joe becoming problematic, his superficial perfect reliability notwithstanding? Somewhere, somehow, something or someone was interfering. Most likely, the interference was serendipitous rather than deliberate. But what if someone, by accident or design, dug too deeply?

Explorations of one thing could point to still other things, other things mandated to remain classified.

Sentinel nodes, like sentinels, stand watch. Their enlargement warns that at a deeper level, something is very much amiss. Will had communicated concern that some outsider connecting with Nick G., Joe Morgan, might begin to figure out what was going on in the deeper levels of Joe's mind, threatening the secrecy of the Program. The pebble of uncertainty tossed by Jeff's casual remarks would generate ever widening ripples, roiling the surface of the Program's tranquil, well-hidden, but far from tiny pond.

Johnson oversaw neutralizing the impacts of unwelcome "somethings," "someones," and "someone elses," smoothing out unwelcome ripples and preventing problems they might create for an organization known as the Glenville-Rodgers Foundation.

SEVEN

Joe Morgan, Nick G., tried to enjoy the wooded view from his apartment window, but his killer headache finally forced him to close the blinds and turn off the lights. He shared a great apartment with Marty Franks, another ex-military college undergrad he'd met through Mike Johnson, a mutual friend. Marty found the place, but needed a roommate to cover the rent. The two men were comfortable with one another and agreed to join forces. Marty spent many weekends away. He had a girl back home in Maryland.

Joe's dark good looks appealed to many coeds. He had as much social life as his classwork and National Guard commitments allowed. Life seemed to be good.

Then, after a few weeks, everything started to go to hell.

Joe hailed from Somerset, Massachusetts. While he was serving overseas, his family perished in a house fire. His hometown no longer felt right to him. Being there became unbearable. Loneliness oppressed him as the holidays neared. In private moments, he wept, hating his own "weakness." He hid his depression from Marty and Mike Johnson, who dropped by on occasion. *How did I handle the holidays last year?* Somehow, Joe just couldn't remember.

A blond girl in one of his classes pursued him. Joe let her catch him. Lying in bed with a girl who really wanted to be with him and made no secret of it was intoxicating. Things began to go better.

Then, they had been making love when she seemed to undergo a transformation. Now he was embracing a pretty raven-haired girl. For a moment Joe thought he knew her. He tried to talk to the girl he thought he saw. He must have called out some name that slipped his mind the moment it passed his lips.

The next thing Joe knew, his lover had given him a hell of a black eye with one solid punch. She burst into tears, jumped out of bed, and followed up her punch with a well-aimed kick to his crotch.

"You bastard! You lousy bastard! You said there was no one else!" she screamed, and stormed out of his life. She never talked to him again.

Alone for the holidays, Joe wandered the deserted campus. He had a brief relationship with a girl as bereft and lonely as he. Mismatched but for their misery, their joyless union was barely better than solitude. Images of the dark-haired girl drifted through his mind. With them he sometimes smelled salt air, or felt sand somewhere in his shoes, or inside his clothes.

Joe Morgan, Nick G., worried about his sanity for nearly half a year before he reached out for help. *And then I get that know-it-all bitch at Student Health. What a dead end! Decorative but useless.* To Joe, Dr. Eve Gilchrist was an audio-animatronic Disneyland robot gone out of whack, her fractured voice track repeating the same gibberish over and over and over. His so-called "doctor" was an exceptionally good-looking and exceptionally empty-headed Barbie Doll, offering nothing more than her bobble-headed beauty.

* * *

Eve Gilchrist steeled herself to follow Ben's advice. She had no illusions that she was always right, but she resented feeling forced. Eve's good looks guaranteed she was rarely confronted no matter what; she usually got away with everything. Her mother, Betty, was a celebrated beauty. Once, after far too many martinis, she counseled Eve, "People just do not like to have beautiful women upset with them, dear. You can usually count on that. But it's better to be right!"

Mother, Eve reflected, *was the sort of person who might have inspired the expression, "in vino veritas"—we tend to tell the truth when we drink too much. Was there a Latin expression that said, "In sobriety is falsehood and deception?" Mother might have inspired that one, too.*

During her first year of training, Eve worked with very troubled inpatients. They generally responded well to her primarily supportive efforts. She could see that while her skills were increasing, usually medication, structure, and the time-limited nature of many crises were more potent factors in her patients' improvement than either she or her psychotherapy.

Now, in the outpatient clinic, things that made her uncomfortable were proving more important than she wanted them to be. Jeff was very fond of her. He tried to bring her along gently. But this Ben Jordan seemed convinced that putting the patient first somehow put the resident and the resident's education first. His way of seeing things made her heart race and her skin crawl.

Eve studied her golden watch. She couldn't delay any longer. She placed the call, praying she'd catch a break and get Joe's answering machine.

No such luck!

"Mr. Morgan? This is Dr. Gilchrist, from Student Health at the U. I hope I can persuade you to come in again, sooner than we initially scheduled."

Eve realized she was racing on, trying to do what she had to do without giving Joe a chance to get a word in edgewise.

"I don't think we really succeeded in clarifying …" *Oh, no! I'm dumping blame on him—"We" when it was all me!*

"Let me start again. I'm not happy with the way our interview went. That's on me. I don't think I came away understanding you well enough to really get a clear picture of where to go next in helping you. I don't want to present your situation to my supervisors when I feel so unclear about things. They have a lot to offer. I want their input. But frankly, if I presented my findings the way they are, I'd look like an idiot, and you wouldn't get the benefit of their best thinking. You know what I mean?"

Joe experienced the faintest hint of hope.

"Yeah. I know what you mean."

"Good. In fact, are you OK with coming in for a double session? I think we have a lot of ground to cover."

"Sounds good." *That,* Joe thought, *was one hell of a turnabout. Maybe … just maybe …*

The call completed, Eve took no comfort from doing the right thing. She wasn't sure that she really wanted to know anything more about whatever was going on in Joe Morgan. What Ben Jordan had taught her about herself was already beginning to work on her mind. *Perhaps,* Eve mused, *I should consider dermatology.*

But then she confronted herself. *No, this is my own stuff! Jeff talks about the countertransferences that reflect distortions that come from the therapist's issues and the countertransferences that come from a whole bunch of normal reactions as well. Ben pushes me to use countertransference as a way of learning things about the patient from my own reactions, not that I usually have any. He wants me to pick up what's beginning to get reenacted between my patient and me. Is my mind telling me I'm afraid to know whatever happened to Joe Morgan? I should really ask Jeff about this stuff, not Ben. I don't want that man mucking around in my head!*

EIGHT

Will's Program extension rang four times and fell silent. Five minutes later it rang again. Will answered on the fourth ring.

"Hey, Will!"

"Yeah, Marty. What's up?"

"He went to a new doctor."

"Who is he? I can ask the docs here to check him out." Will played dumb.

"It's a her, some Dr. Eve Gilchrist at Student Health at the U."

* * *

After a few hours, Johnson reached Will.

"I've been thinking about Nick. If he doesn't want us to know, we have to respect that and find a different way to let him know he's not alone."

"That makes a lot of sense, Mike."

Will translated: Nick G. may be escaping from controls essential to preserve the secrecy of the Program. He was being ordered to reestablish the Program's authority and restore previous levels of training and conditioning.

Defections were fraught with incalculable peril, completely intolerable to Glenville-Rodgers. Whoever meddled with the Program would experience as much discouragement as proved necessary.

Will continued, "In the meantime, I just learned Nick is seeing some Dr Eve Gilchrist over at Student Health. She's a student under supervision. I'll see what I can learn. We want only the best for him."

"Of course. Later."

Eve Gilchrist would become the subject of clandestine surveillance. If necessary, she would be caused to experience discouragement.

NINE

Joe seemed unmoved by Eve's more receptive approach. He trudged to his chair, sat mute with downcast eyes, and seemed to study the floor.

"I looked over my notes from our first meeting. I wasn't pleased with myself," Eve began.

"There were times when I talked too much and listened too little. I'm afraid that I left you with the impression that I was pretty insensitive, and really missed the boat."

Joe looked up briefly before resuming his scrutiny of the floor.

"Given what you told me, and how things went down, if I were you, I would be wondering if someone like me had even the vaguest idea of how to go about understanding you."

Joe looked up. He regarded Eve with curiosity, as if she were a strange and unfamiliar kind of creature.

"In fact, I even wondered if you were wondering if you could ever understand a person like me."

A smile slowly spread across Joe's face. He nodded.

"OK, then. Maybe we should start by looking at what you think I failed to get most completely. Even though we have a double session, we may not come anywhere near to exhausting that list of misunderstandings."

Joe nodded, and laughed a little.

"Yeah. But it's not just you. Sometimes I think it's the whole human race."

"Go on."

"Really?"

"Please."

Joe sighed, and began.

"Has anyone ever told you that they don't think that they're human? Like they kind of look and act like they're human, but really something is wrong? They don't have feelings like other humans? That at times, they feel more like a machine than a person?"

Eve considered the differential diagnosis—schizophrenia, schizoaffective disorder, bipolar disorders, major depression, schizoid personality, schizotypal personality, the autistic spectrum, really bad obsessive compulsives, a good number of the dissociative disorders, especially depersonalization disorder—for starters. Plus, the books Ben recommended stated that under hypnosis, a person could be induced to feel that way. Atypical dissociative disorder? Sure, but giving Joe's vague and nebulous symptoms a vague and nebulous label wouldn't improve the order of the universe.

"Yes. But a lot of conditions can cause that. Sometimes we can only understand the meaning of a symptom by the company it keeps."

Joe smiled. He seemed to relax a little.

"OK, Dr. Gilchrist. I'll tell you about this morning."

This morning? Eve wondered. *What could that have to do with anything?*

She fought off her inclination to redirect Joe to where she thought they should go and uttered words that clashed with her every instinct.

"Don't feel you have to hurry. Don't spare the details. Help me see this morning through your eyes."

"Are you sure that it is worth it?"

"One of my teachers (*May he rot in Hell!*) tells me that his crystal ball is still in the shop, and the damn technicians don't seem to know how to fix it. I can't answer your question today. Maybe sometime down the road. Please, go ahead."

"Well, I got up and made breakfast. So far, so good, you'd think. But I can't even make toast without problems. I caught myself putting sugar on it. What the hell is that about? When I parked on campus and headed over to class, I misread a street sign. It was Edgewood Street, but I thought it said Easton Street. The two seemed to flip in and out. The U library got blurry. Something was making it look higher and thinner. And I smelled salt air. Ow! Goddamn headache! It's a killer!"

"Joe, it sounds to me that we stepped into something your mind may not be ready to deal with. Let's back off and see if the pain settles down."

Eve got Joe to talk about his studies. Fifteen minutes later, he seemed more comfortable.

"I didn't tell you this the first time 'cause every time I mention some injury, everything goes down the brain damage toilet. I'm sick of circling that drain. That can't be the whole thing. There's a lot I don't remember, but it's not just brain damage. I have a mind, damn it!

"I know I suffered head trauma. If I can't fight my way out of this, I won't walk around forever talking suicide. I'll end it.

"A few months ago, I was doing my weekend for the PA National Guard. Still thought my life made sense. There was some weird stuff with women, some things got confused, but basically, things were OK.

"From time to time I've realized that I don't remember my childhood the way other people do. Just a few memories, but those are really clear and vivid. Most folks remember a lot, some vivid, some not. I wondered why I could describe my life as I remember it crystal clear, and everything I remember stands out like a landmark. That's just not normal … Yeah,

I did some reading. I wouldn't have described things like that before I studied some stuff.

"And sometimes, and this is real weird, sometimes, when I'm with a woman, I have trouble seeing her face the way it is."

"Say more."

"You're gonna think I'm crazy. I see another face on top of the face of the woman I'm with."

Eve's stomach grew queasy. She yearned to formulate a question that would move their conversation to another topic, some subject that wouldn't freak her out. She stemmed her own retreat. *The first time I changed the topic it was a good solid clinical decision. I did it to stabilize him. If I do it now, I'm bailing out for me. I can't go back to that Jordan and let him see I ran away again.*

Eve rallied. "That sounds important. I can't promise to get it here and now, but let's begin to work on this together. Is the face that gets superimposed always the same face?"

Joe closed his eyes, concentrating. He put his hands to his temples.

"This is giving me one hell of a headache … Yeah. It's like her hairdo and her age may change, but I'm pretty sure it's always the same woman."

"Can you describe her, in some general way?"

"Well, she has a very pretty face, great smile, dark hair and eyes."

"Anything else?"

"Her complexion would be darker than yours."

"Sounds like a keeper!"

"Ow! Something is zapping my brain. Oh, my God …"

Joe froze in mid-sentence, but continued to breathe normally. Differential diagnoses flew through her mind: *Seizure? Migraine? Stroke? Conversion symptom? Acute catatonia? Dissociative disorder?* Fighting off misgivings and relying on

Joe's relatively normal respiration, she made herself wait and observe.

Tears slowly trickled down Joe's face. Then suddenly he opened his eyes, snapping back to being the Joe she thought she knew.

"That happens when I try to focus on those weird things that flash through my mind. Pain, electric shock sensations, worse pain still. Then I seem to come out of it after a few minutes. Am I crazy?"

"I don't think so, Joe, but you do have a set of symptoms I know very little about—no—almost nothing about. But I have a consultant who's familiar with situations like this.

"Joe, I want to talk to my consultant before exploring the headaches with you, but something confuses me. You talked about real brain damage this time and serving in the National Guard. Both are news to me. Help me see where they fit into the picture."

"OK. This is what happened. I was late heading home from one of my National Guard weekends. To leave the base I had to pass a formation of … Do you know anything about armored battalions?"

"No."

"Well, let's just say, 'big-ass tanks,' OK?"

"Got it."

"I was at a stop sign when someone screamed, 'Stop! Holy shit! Stop!' Next thing I remember, I was in a hospital. A rookie tank driver was getting some extra training. Well, he messed up, jerked into reverse … My airbag deployed right in my face. My car was totaled. I had burns and abrasions on my face, arms, and chest, and headaches that wouldn't stop. They said I just didn't seem to be myself. They said I said all sorts of weird things. I don't remember that.

"Back home I began to get terrible dreams. People were hurting me, electrocuting me, screaming at me. I got flashes of people I didn't know, though somehow they seemed familiar. And that woman I mentioned? Sometimes I got flashes of her, like we were doing normal things together, especially walking among sand dunes God knows where. The doctors said it was my mind's way of representing the trauma of the accident. That's not good enough! The bad stuff expressing the accident's trauma? Maybe. But the girl? What does she have to do with anything?

"My roommate, Marty Franks, comes from money. His family knew some big-shot Harvard neurologist at Beth Israel in Boston. Indian guy. Dr. Charda, Chada—I don't remember his name. He gave me a clean bill of health, brain-wise. That's why I got so pissed off when you wanted to reinvent the wheel.

"When it came to the girl, he put his hand on my shoulder and smiled. 'Joe,' he said, 'sometimes our dream girls are just that—dreams. I hope a real dream girl comes your way soon. That would be nice.' And you know, Dr. Gilchrist, if she looks like the girl who keeps creeping into my head, that would be nicer still."

"Let's hope so, Joe. Let's hope so."

Eve had Joe complete and sign a release form. She faxed a request for his medical records to Beth Israel Hospital in Boston.

TEN

Eve played the tape of her second session with Joe. Ben nodded from time to time, but he neither commented nor asked her to stop the tape.

"Now I really do want to talk a little about diagnosis," Eve ventured.

She took a deep breath. Given the opportunity, Jeff Kane would discourse endlessly about his diagnostic opinions. He seemed to assess a resident's intelligence by how completely the resident agreed with him. But with Ben Jordan Eve would have to risk voicing her own ideas. She took another deep breath, let her body relax slowly as she exhaled, and took the plunge.

"It's an extensive differential. I can say he has post-traumatic stress disorder. But PTSD doesn't explain everything. Could be hysteria, a psychosis, a dissociative disorder, or something organic like a seizure, migraine, or stroke. I considered catatonia, conversion, and bipolar stuff as well."

"How does it break down?"

"There's no firm evidence for organic components, but they're important to keep in mind. Some symptoms suggest problems with reality testing, but the only psychotic diagnosis that really fits is atypical psychosis, where people put hysterical psychosis. The features for the formal psychotic diagnoses, schizophrenia, schizoaffective disorder, and bipolar disorder aren't there. But around here everyone is bipolar these days."

"Right. Bipolar is in. It's like a fashion forecast—this spring, bipolar diagnostic criteria will be worn lower and looser. You're right—psychotic may be an apt descriptor for particular symptoms, but there's no evidence for an actual psychotic condition. Ironically, you can be psychotic without having a psychosis, and you can have a psychosis without being psychotic, like a bipolar patient or schizophrenic in remission.

"So far, so good. Lots of symptoms once listed under hysteria now are linked to the dissociative disorders. Too many symptoms for depersonalization disorder or amnesia to account for them all, and lots of those other symptoms can be part of multiple personality or atypical dissociative disorder. One oddball possibility would be the secondary identity in a fugue falling apart before our eyes. For now, atypical dissociative disorder, probably due to brainwashing. But I wouldn't make that diagnosis yet. Diagnoses have political dimensions. If you make a controversial diagnosis without ironclad evidence, you take the kind of risk I don't want to see residents take. Leave the diagnosis uncertain for now, and wait till we're sure."

"Don't want to commit yourself?"

"For the sake of your education, no."

"Hah!"

"OK, Eve," Ben chuckled. "I'll give you my predictions in a sealed envelope. Don't open it until you're sure yourself. Remember, my job is to help you learn to make the definitive diagnosis, not feed it to you."

Ben typed for several minutes, printed out his opinion, and gave it to Eve in a sealed envelope.

"Now," Ben resumed, "back to the politics of diagnosis. Some things seem plausible, but diagnosing controversial conditions that don't meet gold standard criteria is risky business for a resident. You know the axiom, 'When you hear hoof-beats coming down the hall, don't assume it's a zebra'? With the scoffing these things can stir up, be cautious."

"What about PTSD?"

"What's the trauma?"

"The accident with the big-ass tank?"

"Did it happen?"

"I assume so."

"It probably did."

"But doesn't cover all the bases. His memory problems and misperceptions started months before. Most of the diagnoses we could consider assume facts not in evidence."

"Too true, Dr. G. Imagine presenting this to a case conference: 'The patient is male, probably single, young, but of unknown age and uncertain name. He comes from parts unknown with no reliable history. He hallucinates all over the place and misperceives things in his environment. Findings suggest he's been subjected to extensive mind-control manipulations that most people don't think are possible, and others won't admit exist. First topic for discussion: Who looks crazier? The patient or the presenter?' "

Eve laughed. "Yeah. Not good!"

"Part of my job it to help you learn to diagnose and treat at the highest level. Another part of my job is to teach you how to avoid diving into quicksand. Lay low, get your ducks in a row."

"Politics? Not science?"

"Science has more than its share of politics and dirty tricks. Sometimes issues arise at levels grasped by so few that folks generally assume that the big dog is right."

"I don't want to believe you, but I get it. You didn't say anything about the therapy session itself. Any comments?"

"Everything can be improved. That said, you tracked Joe well, you didn't try to make him think your thoughts, and you responded to his issues, not your own. The session wasn't broke, so I didn't try to fix it. If you want a fine point, 'Sounds like a keeper' said about a girl he's just compared to you in some way could stifle or distort his ability to develop and express any erotic fantasies toward you. If those prove important issues down the road, your words today may prove problematic As kind as they were in context, they may bring you too close to the gal he wants to be with, whether she's an old girlfriend or a dream girl."

"Yeah. I see that."

"But that's a detail, probably no big deal unless you were doing a classic analysis. Just keep it in mind. Overall, it's hard to believe that the same therapist conducted these two sessions. I like what I heard—keep it up. Just remember cases like this always have more surprises in store."

"I said I consult you. Was that wrong?"

"No. You both knew you were confronting issues beyond your expertise, and you said you'd go get help from someone who might have the necessary skills and experience. You avoided the worst error."

"What's that?"

"Immediately moving to transfer Joe to someone with the expertise."

"That never occurred to me. But why would that be so wrong?"

"I'm not saying it would be wrong to transfer him at some point. But he's lost a lot of people and he's just connected with you. Bail out now, and he'll feel rejected and beyond hope, even if you send him to someone more qualified. People get well in relationships. You're off to a good start. I can help you learn, even intervene if need be, but the continuity of a connection is crucial. Expertise can be acquired, but for skills to really be effective, they have to be used in a relationship. And there's another important factor here, indirectly related to that one little point I made earlier."

"What's that?"

"You can scream that I'm a sexist, but it always wounds a man more deeply to be sent away by a beautiful woman than by any other creature short of God."

"But I don't …"

"Trust me on this one. I own a Y chromosome."

ELEVEN

"Jeff, I don't like the idea of Jordan or any of his crew working with this guy."

"Why not, Will? And what do you mean, his crew? It's Eve's case under my supervision. I asked Ben to consult and lend me a hand. This man's problems are *terra incognita* to me. I listened to some excerpts from the last session. He's beginning to open up a little. Eve was doing well. What's your problem?"

"I know. But suppose things get more complicated? If hypnosis was involved in how he was conditioned, someone with a more sophisticated understanding of hypnosis research findings and their implications would be a better consultant than Jordan. I mean, what will Jordan do if he encounters some complex conditioning paradigm?"

Jeffrey Kane liked to run a happy ship. His clinical skills were outstanding, but he discovered very quickly that he just didn't like working with patients. He obtained a prestigious M.B.A., and built his career on administrative expertise and fund-raising skills. Patients were bad enough—Jeff had no stomach for refereeing a pissing match between two truculent professors.

"Well argued. Yet Jordan could complain and say, 'Jeff, if trauma was involved in this patient's conditioning, someone with a more sophisticated understanding of trauma treatment would be a better choice. I mean, what would some researcher do if he encountered overwhelming traumatic material and psychotic regression?'"

"At least let me get a sense of what's going on, so if Jordan needs some help …"

"Will, I rarely question your judgment. But your sudden interest in this case puzzles me. What am I missing?"

Will sat silently for a moment, collecting his thoughts.

Jeff waited. *On a good day*, he mused, *chairing a department of psychiatry is like running a stable of thoroughbreds, all spirited and raring to race. On a difficult day, it's more like keeping a bunch of pitbulls from going at one another. On a really bad day, it's more like herding feral cats.* Was today sliding downhill from thoroughbreds? Could the moment be saved from merciless jaws and savage claws?

"Jeff, you're right," Will began. "Jordan has impressive skills. My concerns are for the best interests of the department. I don't like Jordan. That's no secret. Before your time he created a lot of problems for me. Let's accept that Jordan and I don't play well together. OK?"

"OK."

"Before you arrived at the U, my group received a major grant."

"An impressive grant. It supports a lot of our people."

"That grant came from the Glenville-Rodgers Foundation."

"Glenville-Rodgers doesn't make many grants for psychiatric research."

"True. Just this one."

"Just this one?"

"Right. Let me explain some very complex things in an oversimplified way you may find more useful."

Jeff's neck went tense. Every heartbeat pounded in his ears. If he grasped Will's drift, Will was about to deliver a message obliquely enough to preserve plausible deniability. He would be asked to know something without officially knowing what he knew.

"In addition to the research we publish in mainstream journals, we pursue other projects that never enter the public domain. They are done on contract for particular parties. Those parties are glad to support university programs able to develop such information for them. Are you with me?"

"Yes." Jeff wanted a drink. A stiff drink. At one level this was a calm and affable conversation with a good friend. At another, he could hear the felines hissing. Jeff remembered a scene from a nature show. *Some animal, maybe a caribou, was crossing an ice-covered river during the spring thaw. Raging torrents rushed beneath the ice, eroding it from below even as the sun's warmth melted it from above. That poor beast plunged through the ice and was swept downstream to its doom.*

"This situation came to the attention of Glenville-Rodgers. I don't know how. Think of Glenville-Rodgers as a well-heeled, well-connected patriotic think tank. What concerns them concerns all thoughtful Americans. They shared their worries with me. I want to be able to reassure them. That would be good for the department."

Damned if I'll let myself fall through the ice!

"I think it might be a good idea for me to talk to Jordan."

Good God! Will leaked information to his real masters, and he's bringing their ultimatum back to me. Darymple warned me about crossing Will Rivers. Oh shit! That animal! Is my unconscious warning me not to "cross a river" and get swept to my death ... This guy is scaring me shitless ... Crossing him? I don't think so!

Jeff struggled with himself. Those images proved nothing, but they were waving an enormous red flag.

"I would feel better and more secure here if you did," Will responded.

Jeffrey Kane saw Will out of his office as cordially as he could. Will's remarks left unstated that it was Jeff who would feel better and more secure if he complied. Their unspoken threats, pregnant with menace, felt like a gun pressed to his head.

Jeff knew that Alan Scheflin, a lawyer specializing in psychological and psychiatric issues, especially involving brainwashing and mind control, had spearheaded the use of the Freedom of Information Act to uncover evidence of wrongdoing in secret research projects. In *The Mind Manipulators*, Scheflin and Opton described the cruel and grossly unethical behavior of renowned and respected mental health professionals who betrayed the most fundamental principles of their professions in their research for covert agencies.

In private moments, Jeff Kane dreamed of California. For him, Philadelphia was a just a stepping-stone. In silent prayer, he implored all that was holy in every faith and creed to protect the comfortable, affluent life he worked so hard to cultivate.

Every option he could envision was fraught with risk. Either concealing or revealing the situation could destroy him. Musing, Jeff tried to conjure up consoling images of San Francisco, LA, or San Diego. Even Palo Alto might be his. Nothing could be allowed to tarnish his hitherto unblemished record of success.

When old Bill Darymple had oriented him, he mentioned, so casually that it almost slipped by unnoticed, that Will and his work and the moneys that his research brought in to the department were best handled with a light touch.

"He doesn't react well to interference. There was a problem with one of his people and Will exploded like a volcano. But if you give him room and don't cross him, he will do exactly what you ask. He grinds out papers. He brings in money. He presents all over the world. He puts us on the map. He makes us look good. The pluses outweigh the minuses. Don't kill the goose that lays the golden eggs."

When Jeff arrived in Philadelphia, Will had been incredibly welcoming and supportive. The two quickly became friends. Jeff and his wife looked forward to winter weekends at Will's ski lodge, summer weekends aboard Will's incredible yacht, and fishing trips with Will's lab crew. First class all the way! Once, when Jeff complimented Will on his generosity, Will had laughed, "Well, I have a very rich uncle." Now Jeff read new meanings into Will's words.

Will cultivated a bristly personal reserve, withholding a lot of himself. Claire Kane, who understood people much better than her psychiatrist husband, nicknamed Will "the Black Hole." The Black Hole's fiancée Lou, a dark-haired woman somewhat taller than he, was equally evasive. Her height and reticence earned her the moniker, "Natasha," after the consort of Napoleonic cartoon spy Boris Badenov. *Claire nailed it! She nailed it years before I even suspected there was anything to nail!*

Jeff allowed himself to put the pieces together. Glenville-Rodgers was a front for clandestine funding sources. It would be dangerous to tamper with the arrangement he had inherited.

In Jeff's preferred view of the world, in the natural course of events shit flowed downhill. Jeff took pains to remain perched safely above such fecal avalanches. As chair, he might facilitate or permit their being unleashed upon others down below. But it was downright unnatural for shit to reverse its course, defy gravity, and come roaring back up the mountainside after him!

Ben Jordan, his trusted right hand, had suddenly become a potential liability. Jeff figured Ben might fuss and fume, but knew he had no real authority in the matters at hand. He knew he was a consultant. Ben respected the chain of command. Hopefully, Ben would find a way to take things in his stride.

Weighing all factors, Jeff made his decision. Money (and fear) had spoken. He would cross no rivers. Nothing, and no one, could be permitted to blow up in his face. There was no joy in Jeff's decision, but he would put pressure on Ben.

TWELVE

The Annual Meetings of the American Psychoanalytic Association are held late in the spring in some major American city, anywhere but New York City. Their title is misleading. They are much smaller and far less prestigious than the Association's Winter Meetings.

The Winter Meetings are always held near Christmas in New York City, the capitol of American psychoanalysis. They always take place at the Waldorf Astoria Hotel on the East Side of Manhattan. The Winter Meetings are the big show. Analysts congregate to learn from the luminaries of the profession. Experts from all over the world congregate to interact and be heard. In contrast, many major figures skip the spring Annual Meetings completely, and attendees include the "provincials" of psychoanalysis, those disinclined to make an annual pilgrimage to America's analytic Mecca.

Yet the Annual Meetings are excellent, though less intense. Raymond T. Hawkes, M.D., had never had a paper accepted for the Winter Meetings. He had never had a paper accepted for the Annual Meetings. But this spring he had been called on short notice to substitute for a senior colleague scheduled to discuss an important presentation. Douglas Blake, a spry septuagenarian, took a bad spill spring skiing. Recovering slowly, he was uncertain whether he'd be able to travel. Blake recommended Ray Hawkes be invited to take his place.

Ray was well prepared, and grateful for what he considered an honor. This year the spring meeting was in Washington, DC. As he drove south, Ray actually felt pretty good.

Six months before, things had been different. At the Winter Meetings, his isolation had nearly defeated him. He worked to make excuses to himself, but he had to concede that any reasonable person who took a hard look at his behavior would see that he was trying to destroy himself without making his death appear to be an obvious suicide.

Ben Jordan saved his life. Ray still could not sure whether Ben actually knew what he had done, or whether Ben's friendly gesture accidentally defeated his suicide plan. But now, here he was. He looked around the auditorium, a modern but rather stark venue in a Washington, DC hotel just off Connecticut Avenue, and he felt good.

He actually felt good! Ray had almost forgotten what that was like. Watching the room fill slowly, he remembered another conference room, at the Waldorf Astoria, not that long ago.

Ray had barely been able to stay awake through a three-hour morning panel on some obscure theoretical controversy. Four experts were seated on the dais at the Park Avenue end of the Empire Room. They presented their perspectives and offered learned commentaries on one another's contributions. Inquiries from the audience equaled the presenters' convoluted erudition in their complexity. Perhaps they were meaningful in some alternate universe. Ray had posed a question he thought was relevant. Both the question and the questioner were treated dismissively by those ostensibly in the know.

As the panel came to an end, Ray wondered whether he had been too stupid to appreciate what had been a truly exceptional outpouring of wisdom, or like the little boy in Hans Christian Anderson's fable of *The Emperor's New Clothes*, he had noticed that the great man was bare-ass naked. *Wonder what they did to the little boy?* he mused. *Probably things didn't end with "Happily ever after!"*

Ray gathered up his briefcase and *New York Times*. Lunchtime. Around him people were picking up their programs, coats, notes, or the occasional laptop, and moving slowly toward the single exit. Some returned his greetings, nods, or waves, but no one said anything in response or engaged. He moved over to a cluster of colleagues. A few acknowledged him, but no one invited him to join their group when they moved off.

Asking to come along would have been too much like begging. That he would not do. Besides, many analysts had regular lunch plans at the meeting, annual get-togethers with cross-country friends they rarely saw on other occasions.

Ray stifled a sigh. He had lost all hope for a genuinely positive reception. With practice he'd become an effective fraud. Clutching the *Times*, he muttered, *It's just you and me, Buddy*. He wished he could click into some anesthetized and automatically piloted state rather than struggle to wrench himself painfully into some new mental gear. Battling against his sluggish and grating mental clutch all the way, Ray forced himself to keep his head up.

Striding through the Waldorf lobby with counterfeit confidence, Ray passed clusters of colleagues gathering to meet near its famous clock. He hoped that he looked like he had somewhere interesting to go.

Exiting onto Lexington, he turned right, crossed at the light, and headed east on 49th. As he walked along, he could see people he recognized walking in to one eating place or another, or already seated or being seated near the windows of nearby restaurants. A few waved or returned his waves, but no one beckoned him to join their group.

For the several thousandth time, Ray tried to puzzle out what was going on. What was it about him? What was he doing wrong? Had it always been this way? Or was he so obviously miserable since Emily left him that no one wanted to be caught in the undertow of his pain, the silent screams behind a smile that was a little too fixed, a little too stiff? Had some patients who left his practice spread the word that he was no damn good, absurdly ineffective, or worse, a complete asshole?

Or was it that unspoken scandal that made him a pariah? No good deed goes unpunished. A few years before Jeffrey Kane's arrival, the elder statesman who chaired the department's Ethics Committee retired. After a hiatus of several months, Ray was tapped to succeed him. By then the elder statesman was far away, in a warm climate.

It was a difficult time to become involved in medical ethics. Feminist colleagues and traumatologists had blown the cover off a dirty secret—psychiatrists, psychologists, and social workers had engaged in sexual liaisons with their patients more frequently than anyone wanted to believe. But most mental health professionals still wanted to believe that these transgressions always happened somewhere else.

Ray approached his new responsibilities with diligence and circumspection. He reviewed the old cases and devoted painstaking care to the new charges brought to his attention.

Ray was stunned. His predecessor, a stalwart from the Bill Darymple days, had found grounds on which to dismiss as unfounded every single complaint received by his committee. Among them were accusations of sexual transgressions against the chairman himself! The very person accused of these wrongdoings had simply tossed them aside and buried them forever! A relatively recent report provided convincing evidence that Helen Bidwell, a beloved senior professor, was living in a lesbian relationship with a former patient.

When Ray put these matters before his committee for discussion, attendance at its quarterly meetings plummeted. Stuart Weisel served as acting chair during the prolonged search for Darymple's successor. Ray explained what he'd found to Stuart.

Weisel seemed doggedly determined to be unable to grasp Ray's concerns. He wanted to kick the can down the road. When Ray contended that the foxes had been allowed to guard the hen house, Stuart responded, "You don't want to create a big mess that could blow up in the new guy's face. Why not give him some time to settle in and see whether he thinks it amounts to more than a he said/she said. Let him reach his own conclusions."

Ray accepted Weisel's rationale for the moment. He anticipated Weisel would transmit these concerns to the new chairman, who would want to clean house. Ray waited patiently, his committee effectively on hiatus. Months flew by as the search committee interviewed more than a dozen serious candidates for the chair.

Finally, four acceptable contenders were reinterviewed and ranked. Choice number one led the U on a merry chase, all the while using the U's offer to bargain for a better deal where he was.

Jeffrey Kane was choice number two. He negotiated with the understanding that he could not actually relocate to Philadelphia for several months. An interregnum like this may prove perilous for untenured and out of favor faculty. Interim or acting chairs may issue unpopular decisions that are ostensibly their own, but often reflect skillful exploitations of windows of opportunity for academic bloodletting. An incoming chair may mandate firings, reassignments, and reorganization from afar while remaining shielded from responsibility, however transparently, by the cloak of plausible deniability. Powerful professors eager to settle personal or professional scores below the radar may advocate for actions against adversaries, leaning on an acting chair who may be a co-conspirator, or unable or afraid to stand up to them. Disfavored and deadwood alike risk being purged or reassigned. If they cannot be eliminated, at least they can be marginalized.

Shortly after Jeff accepted the chair, Stuart Weisel called Ray to his office. The acting chair's lugubrious expression would have done credit to a depressed basset hound. Stuart represented himself as profoundly saddened. He told Ray that Jeffrey Kane, the incoming chair, had been surprised to find a person as young as Ray in charge of the Ethics Committee.

The way Stuart Weisel saw things, Jeff Kane was sure to replace Ray on principle, regardless of his merit. Ray would be best served and best protected, Stuart reasoned, if this kind of embarrassment could be avoided. He reminded Ray that his committee had effectively walked out on him. That would not look good if it came to Jeff's attention.

Accordingly, Weisel concluded, a decision had been made to reassign the chairmanship of the Ethics Committee to "someone with more gray hair," the beloved Helen Bidwell. Ray would never learn the identity of those who played a role in his dismissal. It might have involved Weisel himself, Jeff Kane, faculty members who had presented their misgivings about Ray to someone in authority, parties Ray could not even imagine, or inputs from several sources.

Rather than even place such a decision on the record, Weisel suggested that if he were Ray, he would write the acting chair a letter to the effect that he felt ill suited to the Ethics Committee, and hoped that he could be assigned instead to another committee better matched to his talents and interests.

Ray had a wife, two children, an analyst, and a mortgage to support. He was neither well published nor well connected. His career was on the line. Subduing his urge to fight it out, Ray wrote the letter. He listed several other committees on which he would be glad to serve. An hour after he delivered his letter to Weisel, a reply was slipped under his office door.

Ray found that he now chaired a committee he hadn't listed, overseeing the residents' extramural rotations and monitoring their placement in locations remote from the main campus. The letter was long, detailed, and delivered so rapidly that it must have been prepared in advance. His own letter had been pro forma. Appearances notwithstanding, Ray had no voice in determining his fate. He had to admire his tormentors. Their approach minimized the chance he might take what he knew to the state licensing board. If he did, the statutes of limitation on the offenses had long passed, and that delay would be on his head. He still had his appointment, but was so isolated that his prospects for advancement were destroyed.

When Ray and Weisel met again, Weisel reflected that what needed to be done would require no more than one energetic person. To support Ray's new responsibilities, his office would be relocated to the same decrepit building that housed the Residents' Clinic. Ray would report to Ben Jordan, who had been on vacation during this entire debacle, and had never been consulted.

Ray's new office was so small that a vigorous stretch or yawn by a person of his size might cause architectural damage. Unless he stripped the room of virtually all other furniture, his patients would have to sit uncomfortably close to his own chair. He now would be even more isolated from others on the faculty. The easy, friendly conversations throughout the day and occasional congenial lunches with the handful of colleagues who remained friendly were now things of the past.

Matters already had been sliding downhill at home. Emily Hawkes blamed her husband for the collapse of their social life and finances. She had brought two children from her first marriage into the home they made together. Liz and Max had never accepted Ray. Now, they openly despised him.

Ray's wife and kids whined. They couldn't do what other families did, go where other families went, and purchase luxuries other families enjoyed. Liz's plaintive entreaties for one kind of designer jeans after another had already pushed Ray to his limits. Electing a more passive aggressive style, Max filled their dinner conversations with detailed descriptions of the electronic gadgets and games his friends possessed.

Ray sympathized. He had grown up poor. Part of Ray's income package was to be derived from his participation in the U faculty's group practice. In recent years, very few referrals or patient assignments had come his way. His earning power had plummeted, with no signs of recovering.

When Ray was reassigned and his office relocated, Emily's whining stopped. She seemed to become amazingly nurturing and supportive in the face of this latest calamity. A few weeks after the ax had fallen, Emily reviewed Ray's situation with unflinching candor at the end of one particularly painful day.

"You've been tossed away and isolated," said Emily. "It's as if they were afraid you might infect someone with something. They're treating you like a leper!"

For reasons Ray failed to grasp until it was too late, Emily shared this remark with others in their rapidly constricting social circle. It got around. Soon all too many of his colleagues referred to Ray as "the Leper." Much as "Weasel" sometimes slipped out of someone's mouth while talking about Stuart Weisel, "Leper" popped up in Freudian slips when conversations turned to the subject of Ray Hawkes.

The Ethics Committee's work was veiled in confidentiality and secrecy. Only a handful of people suspected that Ray was being punished for raising ethical concerns about venerable and beloved senior colleagues, some of whom were probably the very people throwing him under the bus. Ray himself would be committing a major breach of ethics if he openly voiced his concerns. He could not defend himself. To all outward appearances, he was just a problematic junior colleague whose once-promising career was marching inexorably toward an undistinguished demise.

One beautiful autumn day Ray and Emily planned a date night. They would drive through a nearby preserve to enjoy the peak fall foliage, and have a gourmet dinner at George Perrier's *Le Bec Fin*, Philadelphia's three star culinary paradise. Near noon Emily left word that she had forgotten to go to do something important for their church, something that could not wait. She apologized with convincing sincerity and asked that they postpone their autumn ride till the weekend. But she promised she'd meet him at the restaurant in time for their dinner reservations.

Ray waited for Emily for an hour and a half, nursing a dry martini. He was sure she would arrive at any moment. Ray couldn't reach her by phone. Finally, fearing the worst, he contacted the Lower Merion and Philadelphia Police. No, there had been no accident involving an Emily Hawkes. Neither had local emergency rooms received her. He asked a neighbor to knock on his door. No one seemed to be home. No car could be seen in the garage or the driveway.

Ray lived in Wynnewood, a near suburb. Apologizing profusely to the head waiter, he left 100 dollars for the wait staff, and phoned the Lower Merion Township Police, requesting they meet him at his house. Nightmarish worries and fears tormented him as he drove home.

But what Ray and two policemen discovered when they opened his front door had never crossed his mind. Emily had removed every stick of furniture from their house. Every bit of food, every tool, every cleaning product and necessity—even toilet paper—was gone. Only his clothing remained. The policemen shook their heads and muttered words of sympathy. Then Ray was alone.

The next morning he found that Emily had savaged their bank accounts with the same ruthless efficiency. Since then, his only contacts with the woman he thought was the love of his life had been through her exceptionally aggressive attorney. Ray never learned where she and the children had gone. He finally understood why his efforts to adopt the children had encountered a never-ending series of roadblocks and delays. He was effectively without parental rights. Even if he went to court, the children were old enough to refuse to see him. To friends, neighbors, and colleagues, his wife's leaving and his uncompromising rejection by his children gave credence to the notion that there was something very wrong with Raymond T. Hawkes, M.D.

From that evening on, every meal was a lonely ordeal, and it seemed he was fated to dine solo this lunchtime as well. Between peak autumn foliage and this grim December day he had lost over twenty pounds.

The sirens of ambulances racing by shocked him back to the present. Ray stopped for a light. Searching his memory, he recalled that a drug store nearby sold semi-edible pre-packaged sandwiches. Cardboard bread and unnatural plastic tastes? Or would it be better to skip lunch altogether? Or go back to the Waldorf and pay exorbitant prices for room service? Anything but make apparent to others what was all too apparent to him—He was a leper. No one wants to cozy up to a leper.

He couldn't face the dismal prospect of those drug store sandwiches. He stopped at the next corner, unsure where to turn. A reverie began, orchestrated in a dark minor key. In seconds, it took on a life of its own. *Where on earth would I rather be?* quickly became *There is nowhere else on earth I want to be! Time to get out of Dodge ... big time and forever.*

Somewhere, he heard the rumble of a powerful motor. Without thought or hesitation, he stepped off the curb ...

"Hey, Ray!" A powerful hand grabbed his shoulder and pulled him back before he walked in front a bus, accelerating quickly as it pulled away from the curb.

"You're going the wrong way."

"Pardon?" He recognized Ben Jordan's voice. Slowly, he came back to the here and now.

"You're going the wrong way. The San Martin is on this side of the street."

"The San Martin?"

"They serve cassoulet this time of year."

"What is that?"

"A disgustingly rich French dish with white beans and different sorts of meat. Delicious and heavy enough to make sure you snore through Norman Greenberg's lecture."

"I don't need any help to do that."

"That's the spirit."

Ray sighed. *What the hell did Ben notice? That son of bitch never tips his hand. Does he have my number? Did he reach out to save my life, or just to get my attention?*

"To what do I owe the honor of this invitation? You weren't bored enough by the morning panel?"

"Not quite. Your question offered some promise, but they blew it off. I'm counting on your company to be completely uninteresting and set just the right tone for the afternoon."

"I can do that."

"You overestimate yourself. But I'll tolerate your grandiosity for a while. You'll probably find something interesting to say and I'll be wide awake and have no excuse for missing anything, you no-good son of a bitch."

"Take your chances. Live dangerously."

As they walked, Ray tried to pull himself out of his shell.

"So," Ben asked, "what have you been up to? Last time we really sat down to talk, you were writing a book. How's that going?"

Ray was silent.

"Not good?"

"I got distracted by a thing or two."

At the San Martin, an older analyst was sitting alone. Ben stopped to say hello.

"You probably don't remember me, Dr. Blake. That was a great discussion group yesterday."

"Thanks. A great case presentation always makes the chair look good. José Mendez did a hell of a job. But you know that—you direct a DG of your own."

Ben nodded.

"If you'd like to join us, please do. We were just threatening to bore one another beyond tears."

As simply as that, Ben reached out in a way Ray, certain of rejection, no longer would dare. It turned out that Blake and Ray had a few pet peeves in common. They spent much of the lunch nodding agreements with one another. Thereafter they kept in touch, and even talked about collaborating on a paper. And now, with Blake's fractured femur and blessings, Ray was taking his place on the program, Blake's ironic good wishes ("Break a leg, Ray!") echoing in his ears.

Ray exchanged pleasantries with the man whose paper he would discuss. They took their seats. The colleague chairing the presentation touched bases with both about their introductions.

The chairperson took the podium. Ray noticed Len Liebowitz and Ben Jordan sitting midway back in the gathering crowd. They gave slight waves; Ray responded with a smile and a subtle nod. The chair was concluding his remarks when a familiar figure bustled in and sat immediately behind Jordan and Liebowitz. Ray was astonished to see Stuart Weisel in attendance, and more shocked still when he smiled, waved, and gave Ray a "thumbs up."

THIRTEEN

Unscheduled calls from Marty Franks, Joe's roommate, unsettled Will.

"Got time for a cup of coffee?"

Definitely not good! Will buzzed Jonathan Brewer, his chief research associate. When Ben Jordan filed ethics charges against Brewer, Will was forced to make Brewer first author on some of his own forthcoming major publications to buttress Brewer's defense. Now and forever, Will was relegated to second authorship on some of his best work. He placed the blame for this eternal humiliation at the feet of Ben Jordan.

But fortifying Brewer's standing was essential. As his advocate before the U's board of directors, Will argued it was unthinkable to find Brewer guilty of absurd and unproven allegations in the absence of hard evidence against him. Jonathan Brewer, Will insisted, had become a luminary in his own right, sure to bring additional renown and funding to the U. In fact, Glenville-Rodgers had just given him a grant, administered under the umbrella of Will's funding. Will believed that apart from himself, only Brewer was fully aware of the lab's Glenville-Rogers projects. Neither knew there was a third.

"Jonathan, I have Program business. Please run my subjects today."

* * *

Marty awaited Will at the faculty club. They repaired to an elegant wood-paneled room with many alcoves, the architect's homage to London gentlemen's clubs of another era. An attendant brought coffee.

"Jerry," Will passed a generous tip discretely with a handshake, "we need to concentrate ... tricky grant proposal to think through. Silence and solitude are golden."

Marty began.

"I didn't think we could risk being overheard."

Will nodded. *This better be important!*

"Nick's been pretty shaken up since his second visit to Gilchrist. Things seem OK during the daytime. I can't be precise about when what concerns me got started.

"Come late evening, he gets headaches. He can't concentrate. He can't study. Before the headaches begin, he gets agitated. He stays agitated till he falls asleep. Then, he talks in his sleep."

"Could you make out his words?"

"No. But I know people have a sleep cycle, so I looked up that stuff."

"Good thinking."

"After he woke me up a second time with garbled talk, I figured maybe he'd be clearer if I caught his dreams from the beginning. Since people dream several times a night, about every ninety minutes or so, I set an alarm for myself. But when I went to his room, he wasn't there!"

"What!"

"He didn't come back till after classes the next day. He looking tired, but seemed himself. The next night, I stayed up, nothing happened. The night after that, he was gone before I checked the first time. He was back before breakfast. So far, I'm thinking it's a girl. No worries, right?

"Then, I got to wondering. Sometimes I'm away, off or on other assignments. Sometimes our Nicks need to be followed, but our own Nick would spot us. We swap off. Not often with Nick G. He leads a pretty tame life. But to be sure, I had to know what would happen if he knew I'd be away.

"So I told Joe I had to go on some field trip. Wein covered him, but Nick gave him the slip. I was back before Nick was.

"Will, last month he was gone for a while. When he came back he was miserable. He asked me if I had something stronger than Tylenol for headaches. As per protocol, I went into my stuff and told him that I found some old Percocets. I gave him a couple, and told him I could give him some more if he needed them.

"I'm pretty sure the headaches drove him to call Student Health. Maybe we should get our own docs to give him something."

Will swallowed his rage. More than once, Johnson had warned him, *Will. Remember these are human beings! You treat their complaints as your inconveniences. Some day that will backfire. And what backfires on you backfires on me, and everyone up the line!* Will seethed, *So, I'll act more fucking concerned. What's that sickening bullshit? Fake it till you make it?*

"Marty, that's outstanding work and great initiative. Keep it up and keep me informed. We can't keep them on tight leashes or they'll know they're being controlled and bolt."

They're getting to him! Will thought. *I've got to get them off the case.*

FOURTEEN

Once he had Ben on the phone, Jeff wasted no time in getting down to business.

"I want Dr. Rivers to see Eve's patient in consultation."

"You've got to be kidding, Jeff! This is Eve's case. You supervise her. I consult. If anyone else sticks his nose into this mess, it should be one of us."

"Will has world-class expertise. His insights would be helpful."

"How many patients does Will actually treat?"

"Will? I don't know."

"I've been here longer than you, Jeff. He hasn't seen a patient for over twenty years. He's never been licensed. Putting this patient in Will's hands supports practicing without a license."

Jeff cursed to himself. *That slipped by me. No! I can spin it as research.*

Ben proposed a compromise. "What if Eve presents the case to him for his input?"

"Will really believes his research protocols could offer some helpful insights."

"What protocols? I read all of his stuff. No way! Unless he's doing some stuff I don't know about."

"Of course he is. What else is new?"

"Well, you must have some idea ..."

"He runs his own ship."

"No oversight? That's not how you do things!"

Not usually, Jeff consoled himself.

"The subject is closed. Set it up."

"You're asking me to do something unethical."

"You're out of line. Why do I put up with you?"

"You know we can't play games with this patient! He's too vulnerable. You're proposing something with no clear therapeutic purpose that could wreck his ongoing treatment! If this guy experienced hypnosis or something like that in a hurtful context, he's safer beginning with someone who won't do anything aggressive right off the bat. Beginning with a modality he may associate with bad stuff is just plain wrong! Dashing into complicated medical situations to do things without therapeutic merit has been wrong since the time of Hippocrates. You're proposing illegal and unethical behavior."

"Don't go there, Ben! Will's work can be understood as research."

"Research? Research with no hypothesis to test, no protocol, no project, no informed consent, no meaningful assessment of the cost/benefit ratio of what's being proposed, no license, and no Institutional Review Board or Human Subjects Safety Committee approval? Bullshit! This turns Hippocrates' first principle upside down. Remember? 'Firstly, do no harm.'"

"Ben, you're preaching like the Leper!"

"I've never heard this kind of crap from you before! Whatever is going on, I don't want any part of it. Neither do you. I've always stood behind you. But this? No! Not at the expense of patient care."

"I could fire you, Ben."

"Fair enough. I won't work for some misguided apologist for Will and Jonathan 'See you later, perpetrator' Brewer. When the Jeffrey Kane I know and respect comes back to his senses, swears off whatever funny shit he's been smoking, and returns to his duties as chairman, I'll be glad to be back on staff."

"I won't stand for this insubordination. Lots of folks would kill for your job. Set up this consultation by noon tomorrow or you're fired. We've been friends a long time, so you have the option of submitting a letter of resignation before I fire you. Do you hear me, Ben?"

The line was dead. Somewhere in the course of Jeff's tirade, Ben Jordan had hung up on his friend and chairman.

Just as well, Jeff tried to convince himself, *more than one way to skin a cat.*

FIFTEEN

"So, I wind up wondering ... Is this really possible? Is this wild speculation or is it real? And if it is real, what does it mean that we are doing it? By we I mean America. I mean, this is America! Is this happening here?"

Eve fidgeted with her heavy gold necklace. *The fingering of secular prayer beads by a devout modern fashionista,* Ben reflected. *She's really upset!*

"My dad's been a diplomat and ambassador all over the world. I'm sure I was shielded from a lot of things, but I'm used to the Americans being the good guys. Dr. Kane ordered me to schedule this interview right away. I'm sorry, Ben. I don't understand."

"So, that SOB wormed his way past Jeff? Too bad." Once Ben had wondered whether Jeff's interest in Eve was inappropriate. Over time he appreciated that Eve was Jeff's protégé, nothing more. *Eve could get caught in a loyalty conflict that could mess up their bond. No small matter for her career. Time to step in.*

Eve's efforts to hide her distress collapsed. "I wish I understood. Dr. Kane has always been ... Well, he impresses me. He's very smart, very dedicated, and he's been a good teacher and mentor. I'm very comfortable with him. You ... Honestly, you take some getting used to."

Eve struggled to say what she needed to say and still keep things smooth and safe.

"You're a very different kind of person. Frankly, I still feel uncomfortable with you. But I know ... How can I say this ...? You are incredibly bright and incredibly dedicated. I'm not sure I understand where you are coming from, but even though I don't want to agree with you, something doesn't add up. I just don't understand this big deal research protocol Will has in mind. There's nothing like what he's talking about anywhere in the literature."

"Hell of a loyalty conflict!"

"Yeah."

"Look, Eve. We—that means Jeff and me—not you and me—we have to get you out of the middle, and keep you out. I can't allow any resident to take a hit over a difference of opinion between two senior people. Don't even try to talk yourself into defending one person to the other or trying to make everybody happy. Good people get messed up or worse trying to break up a fight.

"Will is a shit for doing whatever he's doing. You have to let the big dogs either fight it out or grow up and get sane about it. Jeff is a good man. I like him. I respect him. But something is making him run scared. He's better than this.

"So, here's what you are going to do. Follow Jeff's instructions. To the letter."

"But, what about ..."

"My battle. Mine, not yours!"

"What will you do?"

"First, I won't throw you back in the middle by telling you what I plan to do. Second, if Will wins, and he might because he brings more grant money into the department than anyone else, it would be very instructive for you to be present when he sees your patient, both to support your patient and to enhance your own professional growth. Will really can't keep you out, because Jeff's promoting this as a wonderful learning opportunity, and you're here to learn. Right?"

"That's the party line."

"Precisely. So, how could you miss an opportunity like this? We can't let Will hog all the learning."

Eve watched Ben's expression turn grim.

"You are about to see the best of the best in action. Observe carefully. Take good notes, and write down as much as you remember later. Document anything Will does that don't seem to be part of a research protocol, anything about the way he relates to his subject."

"Subject?"

"Yeah. We call people we're trying to help our 'patients.' We call people we're studying but not directly trying to help our 'subjects.'"

Eve nodded. She rose to go, then stopped and turned back to Ben.

"Just to play devil's advocate—Why do you distrust Will so much?"

Ben hesitated.

"I don't mean to put you in a difficult spot," Eve apologized.

"You may not mean to, but you have a distinct gift for it."

They both laughed.

"OK. The way Will tried to pump you for information was dishonest enough to establish him as a flagrant liar, but that's the tip of the iceberg.

"I was filling in at Student Health back in Darymple's time. An undergrad woman presented with acute anxiety. Her story upset me."

Ben studied Eve's expression.

"Should I go on?"

Eve nodded.

"She was a subject in a study in Will's lab, norming a new hypnotizability scale. Know anything about that kind of thing?"

"No, I don't."

"Well, a hypnotizability scale is really a series of challenges or suggestions. The way the subject responds to each yields an item score, and all the item scores give an overall guesstimation of hypnotizability and suggest which particular hypnotic skills or talents are most developed in that subject—like the ability to see vivid imagery with eyes shut and with eyes open, the ability to block sensations, and so on. With me?"

Eve nodded.

"So this experimenter was administering the scale when she began to feel something she shouldn't be feeling. She opens her eyes. The experimenter was fondling her breasts."

"No!"

"Assholes who earn advanced degrees don't become better people. You just have to call them 'Dr. Asshole.'"

"But don't people in trance form false memories, confabulations, stuff like that? Will studied those things."

"True. Though I doubt that this scale had any item suggesting a hallucination that the experimenter is feeling up the subject. But possibility doesn't mean probability, and probability shouldn't be inflated into unwarranted assumptions, and into foregone conclusions."

"But doesn't that go both ways?"

"Sure. I don't know for sure what happened in that room on that day. The woman was devastated. I reported the incident through appropriate channels. I thought Will would support efforts to get to the bottom of things and take steps to discipline anyone who behaved badly.

"That's not what happened. Will met with Darymple and pitched a fit. He insisted that the student was a superlative hypnotic subject who probably had developed a strong emotional reaction to the experimenter facilitated by trance, which is great for intensifying emotion and precipitating rapid transference reactions. He quoted studies that supported his version of things, vouched for his man, and offered to meet with the woman personally and straighten out any misunderstandings."

"What happened?"

"Will met with the student and her parents. He convinced the parents that their daughter must be mistaken. When the student held her ground, Will convinced them she was paranoid. He empathized with their suffering in supporting their mentally ill daughter. He offered to recommend a good therapist."

"And?"

"A happy ending. The ethics charges went nowhere. The student attempted suicide and was hospitalized at Sheppard Pratt in Baltimore. She never returned to the U. She has no relationship with her parents and siblings. They're academics and baby academics. Trusting the gods of the U, they betrayed her and still think she must be crazy."

"How do you know the follow-up?"

"Don't expect an answer."

"Do you think she was abused?"

"I couldn't swear to it in court as a matter of fact. But clinically, something bad went down. I tend to believe her."

"Tend to?"

"The rat did it. One piece of shit protected another piece of shit."

Ben paused. "There is something else you should know. That new scale? It's never been presented or published."

"What does that mean?"

Ben sighed. "It could mean the research is still going on. Maybe one question just led to another. Maybe the work went nowhere and they cut their losses ... It's unlikely that they ran out of subjects or money, not with big grants and participation in an experiment mandatory for all introductory psych students.

"Developing a hypnotizability scale is a major enterprise, a lot of work. Hypnosis research is demanding. It has very high standards. Any new instrument not only has to be studied in its own right. It has to be normed. You have to see what healthy subjects do and report when they take it. You could start with a population of convenience, psychology undergrads, the human lab rat …"

"Easy enough."

"That can tell you something about reliability—for that group. Reliability tells you that you can count on the test to do the same thing over and over. But whether what an instrument does reliably means anything … That's the realm of validity, and several important kinds of validity have to be explored. But you know all of this … or you should. Being you, you do. It's useless to have something that reliably generates meaningless nonsense, no matter how good it looks. So, you have to establish that what it measures is meaningful, useful, and the same as or close to the construct of hypnosis as measured by other tests already considered valid. What it does and what it shows would have to be compared with the scales already out there, tried and true ones like the Stanford Scales, by Hilgard and Weitzenhoffer, like the Harvard Scales, by Orne and his colleagues. This demands an enormous amount of work. You publish it. You share it with the scientific community. Coming up with a new, improved, and demonstrably valid hypnotizability scale just might give you bragging rights for the next quarter to half a century. That's no small potatoes.

"Will says he's been on this project for years. But I've been at the annual meetings of both SCEH and ASCH … Sorry, that's the Society for Clinical and Experimental Hypnosis and the American Society of Clinical Hypnosis. There have been no reports or discussions of such a scale, and no buzz among academics about Will's new scale. And there would be—for sure."

Eve fingered her necklace. "What then? All that effort for nothing? That makes no sense either."

"Well, you're right if things are as they seem. But consider this: Will does a lot of work in social psychology. In one common strategy, you misdirect the subject about the true purpose of the research you're doing. Like you run an experiment, but during the experiment someone else is introduced or blunders into the situation, does or says something, and quickly leaves. The real purpose of the study is to explore the impact of that intrusion or the questions you can ask about the intrusion and/or intruder, but to the subject, it seems like the intrusion is just a glitch in the real study."

"Are you saying that that girl had been participating in what was really a completely different experiment and had no idea about what was going on?"

"Right. Perhaps Will does do the kind of research he says he does. But what else is going on? I checked out the foundation that's supposed to be funding him. I found nothing. Bill Darymple told me that it keeps a low profile by design. You can't apply for their grants. Their directors try to find the next generation of rising stars, and back them."

"Isn't that plausible?"

"Completely. That's the way the MacArthur Foundation works."

"The genius grants?"

"Yep. But the MacArthur people don't try to hide beneath a rock. They just state their policy and go on about their business."

"You said that to Dr. Darymple?"

"Sure."

"And?"

"He said it wasn't worth worrying about. That's just how they do things."

Pieces of an ugly puzzle were clicking into place in Eve's mind. She slumped back into a chair, feeling nauseous. Finally, she found her voice.

"I don't like what I'm thinking."

She lifted her eyes. Ben was looking off into space, his face grim and stony.

"I like what you're thinking. I don't like what I think that bastard is doing."

Eve had seen that look once before. "Uncle Buck," the Marine sergeant assigned to guard her, was leading the Marine detail escorting embassy dependents to a military air base for evacuation. That night a man she knew as a laughing joker was very different, grim, and ready to defend her family with his life.

Something seemed very strange and very wrong. And it seemed to bring out a similar dark, determined, and somewhat frightening side of Ben Jordan.

SIXTEEN

Joe Morgan, the Program's Nick Gregorides, was a highly valuable asset. All programmed Nicks or operatives in other name-coded protocols received certain training in common. However, individual differences were often exploited to create uniquely qualified agents.

Nick C. possessed an astonishingly retentive memory. He was educated to apply it for the Program's purposes. The extremely handsome Nick W. was groomed to enhance his seductive prowess, facilitating his ability to extract information from both genders.

Nick G. was a stealthy warrior. The not-quite-good-enough football player and scholar was a dead shot, expert with edged weapons, and becoming a formidable martial artist. He would be a specialist in infiltration.

Program operatives had to be highly hypnotizable. Protocols were developed for each to create states of mind with useful attributes and carefully calibrated degrees of awareness of one another. Clinical multiple personality cases initially develop different identities with their own individual purposes, motivations, and memories to defend against overwhelming childhood experiences. In contrast, states created by the Program were without motivation or direction, designed to keep their specific functions latent until called upon. The exception was that each operative had been trained to create an overseer charged with keeping whichever function was currently activated on what the Program considered the straight and narrow.

Peter Souza was dedicated and patriotic. Program associates in the military recommended recruiting him. An intelligence platoon had been created within the headquarters company of a general involved with Glenville-Rodgers. Its personnel were trained in both spy craft and advanced combat skills. Those with promise received more specialized training still.

Once discharged and employed by the Program, their hypnotic talents for tolerating contradictory perceptions and thoughts without experiencing distress, for confabulating over omissions, and for both positive and negative hallucinations were carefully cultivated. After six months of daily training, a man like Nick G. could stare at a blank wall and see whatever he was told to see, and transform that into an ongoing movie-like series of perceptions as vivid as external reality. Nick G. learned to look at something right in front of him and either not see it at all, or to project a completely different image upon that something. Since what people see, they generally store in memory as autobiographic events, gifted subjects could be led to incorporate instructed scenarios into their autobiographic memories of what they had experienced.

After a full year of this intense training, Nick G. could be taught a version of his life that in most respects was very much like his own, but the identities of places he had been and people he had known could be altered, slowly and gradually. While the gist of something might be preserved, details could be manipulated to diverge further and further from the details of the life he had previously lived. Memories of his actual hometown could be replaced by memories of another. His Army service could be replaced by recollections of when he had been a Marine.

And at the same time, with aversive conditioning via electric shocks, and with positive and negative induced hallucinations, Nick could be caused to distance the truths of his life far from his newly created identity. In fact, if he came anywhere near locations or individuals from his actual past, he would begin to suffer intolerable migraines and experience electric shocks tormenting extremely sensitive parts of his body. But Nick was led to know that by using his skills to make forbidden memories vanish, comfort could be restored.

After a year and a half, Nick could be placed in the deepest possible trance and caused to understand that his parents, his brothers, his sisters, and the girl he loved had perished. He now could "remember" attending their funerals in the town he now believed had been his hometown. He was taught that returning to the hometown he had been taught to think was his own would be too painful to bear. A thousand little things might catapult him into pain and grief, into anguish that would end only when he left the area. Should Nick find himself in his actual hometown, he would not recognize anyone, no matter how close to him they had been. Over and over, he was taught that it was best to move on, to accept the need to start over.

Nick G. was a code name. Peter Souza was trained to elaborate Joe Morgan as an alternate identity. He learned Joe's life story as if it were a role he would play. He was rehearsed in that role, over and over, month after month. Keen and painful experiences of the loss of loved ones, different for each identity, were imposed upon both the Peter Souza and Joe Morgan identities.

Peter was helped to understand that he would be far more effective if he withdrew his attention from himself as Peter Souza. With nothing to go back to, better to become Joe Morgan! Both systematic reinforcement of the Joe Morgan identity and extensive aversive conditioning to distance him from positive connections to the Peter Souza identity became cornerstones of his training.

Still under the guise of helping Joe Morgan, codename Nick G., enhance his expertise, and beyond the efforts to manipulate his core identity, many months of training were dedicated to installing the sense of another entity. Ares, named for the Greek god of war, was created to be his rather sadistic mentor, to administer ongoing orders and ongoing aversive stimuli by conjuring up recollections so painful that they were indistinguishable from the original experiences of both historical and suggested events.

Joe/Nick would be asked a question. But if the answer involved something his trainers wanted to banish from his conscious mind, the trainer would call upon Ares to administer genital shocks. Soon the mere mention of Ares caused Peter/Nick to experience genital shocks, much as Pavlov's dogs, exposed to the pairing of food and a bell tone, came to salivate at the sound of a bell.

Merely the experience or hint of Ares's presence usually brought Joe/Nick in line. Failing this, Ares barked orders that would be heard in the privacy of the mind, or would play the role of the trainer in the mind's own inner theatre and experience himself administering the shocks Joe/Nick actually felt. Here, too, what was visualized became stored as actual autobiographic memory. Joe/Nick accepted the trance logic of the situation. That is, he left unchallenged two perceptions that were incompatible with one another—Ares was simultaneously a suggested structure and function within his mind and a potent entity with a mission of its own that possessed the capacity to rule him and the power to torment him to the point of anguish, despair, and abject submission.

After the domination of Joe/Nick was well established, all self-references to the former Peter Souza identity were brutally discouraged by Ares, who reinforced the trainer's instructions whenever Joe/Nick was awake. Only then, when the trainers were confident that they could eliminate anything they wanted to remove from Joe or Nick's awareness, would the program create Mars.

Mars became the repository of Joe/Nick's martial arts skills and specialized lethal knowledge. Mars was to carry out missions assigned by the Program. Ares systematically suppressed tendencies in Mars toward softer or tender emotions.

Finally, trainers induced Seth, an entity named for the Egyptian god of evil and chaos. Seth remained hidden behind powerfully reinforced negative hallucinations. Responsive only to trainers designated by the Program, Seth's task was to create whatever distortions of perception might be necessary to keep other parts in order, or on track to complete an unpalatable assignment.

Mike Johnson wished he didn't have to keep looking over Will's shoulder. Will, his gifts notwithstanding, was too self-centered, grandiose, and angry to best use his talents for the Program. Johnson managed to contain his own temper in Program business and expected no less from his associates.

Johnson was the best there was at what he did, and knew it. Others were more talented, more original, and more creative. But they were too full of themselves. Johnson realized these others relied on their impressive personal strengths and charisma to work quite rapidly. Many students of hypnosis idealize gifted clinicians and researchers who devise creative and dramatic approaches that achieve rapid results after so many others have tried and failed. Their efforts often appear to be magical.

Get enough dazzling results, and you can begin to believe your own press, Johnson observed. *Everybody wants to be Milton Erickson. They forget how much hard work Milton Erickson put into what could seem to be so swift and amazing. He was wise enough to advise others to be themselves, not to try to be Milton Erickson. Others were stupid enough to try to be Milton Erickson.*

Johnson's predecessors and competitors designed their approaches to get results quickly. Instead, Johnson developed regimens of prolonged intensive and extensive training for each and every skill to be acquired. Where others had considered less than a dozen repetitions quite sufficient, Johnson insisted upon thousands. He made more extensive use of both positive reinforcement and aversive conditioning than the others. His results were the best, but the most costly.

When budgetary axes fell, weaker experimenters seemed like bargains by comparison, and survived. Johnson's funds were slashed so abruptly that he had neither resources nor time to help his special operatives become safe to rejoin the ranks of the military or blend into the civilian population.

He was packing up his desk when a man far above him in his chain of command paid a visit.

"Well, when life closes one door, it often opens another."

Johnson wanted to strangle him.

"Purse strings are tighter and tighter in all the intelligence communities. Let's face it. You are the best, but you are not now and never will be the lowest bidder.

"Your work has impressed some pretty influential people here and abroad. There is interest in taking it into the private sector, with the understanding that it will never be used against the United States or its allies."

A few productive meetings later, a chauffeur-driven limo brought Mike Johnson down a long driveway to the campus of the Glenville-Rodgers Foundation. He was ushered to a luxurious office suite. He saw his real name on its hardwood door, along with the words, "Vice President."

Johnson reached out to the men who had worked with him. His generous offers brought the majority under the Glenville-Rodgers umbrella. The remainder disappeared. Members of the special platoon joined the project upon completion of their enlistments at salaries too generous to refuse, or seemed to vanish.

In short order, a network of scholars at many of the world's best universities was established to pursue research funded by Glenville-Rodgers. Only a handful knew that their projects were part of a grand design, skillfully orchestrated to keep its researchers disconnected from one another. Without inside information the most brilliant scholars would be hard-pressed to infer the overall objectives of Glenville-Rodgers's Program.

SEVENTEEN

Seated behind a one-way mirror, Johnson could see Joe Morgan/Nick Gregorides seated in a chair, a blanket covering his body. Wires, electrodes, and the straps binding Joe were hidden. Despite the paraphernalia, Joe and Will chatted amiably.

Johnson postponed activating his earphones. Will's work made him want to scream or slap him silly. He'd counseled Will to use a more conversational style, but Will's verbalizations remained formulaic and mechanical, as if he were plagiarizing the dialog of terrible sci-fi movies. *Oh, well! The powers that be are infatuated with his credentials and wary of his temper.*

Will led Nick into trance, working slowly, making efforts to be kind and gentle. One after another, Will called upon the various states of mind. When each in turn was predominant, he turned on a tape player and played the same sequence of words. Each sequence was followed by powerful electric shocks to Nick's head and genitals.

"Henry."

BZZZZ! Nick's body seemed to be trying to leap through the restraints, up into the air. "Henry" was Peter Souza's middle name. This intervention was among Will's efforts to disconnect him from every aspect of his identity, and from Prince Henry the Navigator, an iconic figure in Portuguese history, and the source of his middle name.

"March King." Again a buzz. Nick's body jerked, seeming to jump against a powerful tether. John Philip Sousa was "the March King." Turning Nick off to the mere mention of a famous person of Portuguese descent whose surname was similar to his own weakened other links to his actual past, and undermined associations to his grandfather, Philippe Souza. *Nice touch, Will!*

"Madeiros." Maryellen Madeiros was Peter Souza's high school girlfriend, the girl he'd hoped to marry, the girl he'd been told had died in an auto crash. Affection and caring are difficult adversaries. Assassination instructions are vulnerable to disruption if the assassin suddenly remembers his intended victim is the love of his life. The shocks associated with Maryellen Madeiros were administered at a dangerous level of intensity. If something went wrong, Joe was out of luck. Will would never summon someone as sharp as Bobby Gray to the scene. If things went sour, Jonathan Brewer would lose Joe's body in the New Jersey Pine Barrens, one of organized crime's celebrated cemeteries.

After Will worked his way through the remainder of Nick's aversive conditioning module, he took a break. Nick seemed oblivious to what he had just endured.

* * *

As the next part of Nick's training began, Johnson's already sour expression moved toward frank disgust.

"Ares?"

"Affirmative."

"Problems to call to my attention?"

"Affirmative."

"Report."

"Intensifying emotional forces regarding pre-training life and involvements. Instructions awaited."

"Elevate to and maintain highest possible deterrent efforts. You will clear the way for Mars and Seth if necessary."

"Understood."

"Good-bye then, Ares."

Will was instructing Ares to give Joe hell for any Peter-like intrusions, and protect actions by Mars or Seth from interruption by Joe or Peter moments.

Short and sweet, but oh, so mechanical. Johnson grimaced. *Is Will working to make things more impersonal to create another layer of distance between the subject and what might upset this programming, or is he just an insensitive prick? Well, they're not mutually exclusive.*

Will accessed Mars.

"Are you mission-ready?"

"Affirmative given above."

Mars was able to hear conversations involving Ares or Seth if they involved his own areas of endeavor. Otherwise, he remained oblivious. It was imperative that Mars remain completely cold and detached from potential victims. Mars understood that if he had to act, powerful forces in the mind would be allies and assistants, clearing his way.

"In the days to come, Nick will appreciate more and more that Dr. Gilchrist, Eve Gilchrist, and Dr. Jordan, Ben Jordan, are dangerous and will have to be eliminated from his life. Others will discourage them. Should that fail, you will find the optimal circumstances to effect their termination."

"Query! This contradicts previous orders. Please confirm the change."

"Affirmative."

"Code?"

"Omega Omega Omega."

"Restating orders: Await results of discouragements. If discouragements fail, terminate Eve Gilchrist, Doctor, and Ben Jordan, Doctor, under optimal circumstances."

"Affirmative."

* * *

Will stretched and paused. He walked around a bit, and then sat down to complete his efforts.

"Seth?"

"Affirmative."

"How are things proceeding?"

"Level one substitutions, Level one frequency." Seth was causing Joe to misperceive people and places a few times a week, and disrupting any intimate ties he tried to create.

"Are you prepared to raise substitution and frequency levels?"

"Affirmative. Details requested."

"Maryellen Madeiros/Street Prostitute 75%. Dr. Gilchrist/ Maryellen Madeiros/Street Prostitute 50–60%. Dr. Jordan/ Adolf Hitler/Armed Arab Terrorist 50–60%."

"Affirmative. Onset?"

"About five or six minutes into Nick's next session with Dr. Gilchrist."

No! Johnson wanted to scream. *No! No! No! Your hatred for Ben Jordan fucks up your judgment! Degrading Peter's old girlfriend into a whore, confusing Gilchrist with the degraded image of his old girlfriend—Those probably will work. But linking Ben Jordan to images that would piss off a Jew but may be meaningless to non-Jew? In the unlikely event that the Souza family were hidden Jews who'd kept their faith secret from the Inquisition to the present day, that move is pure genius! If not, it's just plain stupid! But jerking Will's chain in the middle of an operation is unsound policy. This will have to do.*

Johnson forced his attention back to Will's procedures.

"Seth?"

"Affirmative."
"Time limited command."
"Proceed."
"Next interview?"
"Yes."
"Palm down, help him see the evil, state the evil."
"Understood."

* * *

Before dehypnosis Will suggested that upon arriving at a bar with Marty, Joe would recall that he'd bumped into Marty Franks and they'd already had a few drinks. Nick would even feel their effect.

Marty intercepted Joe outside the lab and took him to a crowded dive near campus. After a couple rounds, Marty told Joe it was probably time to go home because he looked wasted. Joe had only had a beer and a half, but suddenly he felt kind of tipsy. Home they went.

At a more upscale bar off Rittenhouse Square, Will congratulated himself on his night's work until Johnson warned him he was getting too loud. Johnson switched the subject.

"This fellow Ben Jordan is Jewish, you know?"

"Yeah."

"What kind?"

"Circumcised, I guess."

"No, seriously. It will help me to understand his thinking. Is he Orthodox, Conservative …?"

"I have no idea."

"Well, what about where his people are from?"

"No idea."

"I assume Gregorides thinks he's Greek Orthodox."

"Yes. We brought in someone special for that part of his reconditioning."

"But his original religion was …"

"Catholic. Portuguese are Catholics."

"Always?"

"Always," Will replied.

"Yeah! What else would they be?"

Will, Johnson thought, *You just love yourself too much to rise to the top. I'm beginning to think you're a liability!* In the Program, those who worked together were recused from evaluating one another. They just reported facts. Other Glenville-Rodgers research suggested that past conflicts over subjective aspects of evaluations impaired teamwork during missions. Angry armed men can be darn ingenious in arranging permanent paybacks. *When this is over, you and your work will be reviewed by someone who's had no contact with you. Let's see how your egotistic bullshit flies if we bring some overseas hard-ass into town.*

EIGHTEEN

Eve arrived early to Will's lab. His secretary surprised her. She was a lovely, articulate, and well-dressed Englishwoman in her late thirties. *She looks like a heavy-hitting professional or exec. Where on earth does Will get the money to hire her?*

Eve quickly learned she was a professor from the London School of Economics, on sabbatical while her barrister husband completed the U's international law program. Collaborative research with professors at Penn's Wharton School occupied most of her time. Her part-time work in Will's unit meant nothing to her, but American prices were unexpectedly high, so …

When Joe arrived, he barely responded to Eve's greetings. They sat in uncomfortable silence. *What's going on? Some turnabout!*

At the appointed time Will ushered them to his office, unusually large and luxurious by U standards. Ben had briefed Eve on the demanding requirements for forensic hypnosis, among which were videotaping complete views of both interviewer and interviewee. He had asked her to be alert for anything that fell short of forensic standards.

"If Will wants to show his work is squeaky clean," Ben had said, "here's his chance."

Will's video camera was positioned to capture Joe's face and upper body. Eve tried to contain herself. *This set-up won't record Joe's lower body or Will's behavior. Joe could be half-naked and Will could be pointing a gun at Joe off camera, and no one would be the wiser.*

Will explained that this interview would not be directly therapeutic in nature. Instead, it was designed to explore and learn things that might prove helpful for his psychotherapy. After this preliminary interview, Joe would receive several tests of hypnotizability, but first it was important to get to know him without the intrusiveness of formal testing. Will reviewed the concerns necessary to obtain informed consent for the upcoming interview. The consent form signed, Will turned on the camera and began.

As he moved carefully and respectfully from one subject to another, Will's interviewing skills were impressive. Will explored Joe's childhood in Somerset, Massachusetts. His early years were pleasant and uneventful. Early on, athletics became the center of his life. Joe hadn't taken school very seriously.

Just before Joe went off to college, he learned that his sweetheart had been promiscuous. The girl he wanted to marry was no more than a slut! That messed up his head. Unable to concentrate in college, Joe dropped out and joined the Marines. That slut died in an auto accident while he was overseas. Good riddance! Now he was back, pursuing a college degree.

This is news to me! He didn't tell me any of this! Time and time again Eve was shocked by contradictions between the history Joe was presenting to Will and what he had told her.

When Will asked Joe about his National Guard experiences, Eve relaxed. She thought she already knew what Joe would say. Her attention focused on Will.

"I was leaving late. I was behind this tank …"

Will suddenly lowered his right hand below waist level, palm down, parallel to the floor.

"... when I began to remember that fuckin' slut. I got so angry that I lost track of where I was. It wasn't till the airbag exploded ..."

Eve looked back to Will. His right hand held a pen poised over his clipboard.

Minutes later, Will asked Joe about his goals in treatment.

"Well, I'm really confused about who I am. I want to figure out what happened to me."

"How has Dr. Gilchrist tried to assist you?"

"Well, so far all she's done is ask me to tell her about my life. We're just beginning."

"And I wish you the best in that project, Joe. But it does cause me some concern."

"Concern?"

"Why, yes. You know, Joe, memory is not a tape recorder. It's not like we push the right button on the right place on the right tape, and out comes your past."

"No?"

"No. As a matter of fact, most responsible scholars are very cautious about trusting memory. Since it's not just there like a tape, when we go for memory we may get a confusing grab-bag of fact, fiction, and encouraged imagination."

"So what comes up may not be true?"

"Yes, indeed. That's why many of us who are true scientists worry about whether therapies designed to uncover the past, however good their intentions, may cause more harm than good."

Eve saw Will extend his hand, palm down.

"Well, shit!" Joe exploded, his face becoming red. "So this treatment could really screw up my head! Is that what you're saying?"

"Not just me, Joe. Many of us worry about things like this. Unfortunately, many therapies today do dwell on the past. Psychoanalysis and hypnosis are used to explore the past ... "

"If they are so … oh, I don't know … bad … why do therapists do them?"

"Well, those schools of thought have been around a long time, and it's hard to change people's minds. When therapists have used an approach for a while, it becomes part of the way they view the world."

Eve made a bet with herself that Will's hand would go out, palm down. She won her wager.

"Are you saying that Dr. Gilchrist and whoever her supervisors or whatever …? Are you saying that they are doing bad treatments?"

"Well, perhaps I spoke too strongly …"

Eve glanced quickly. Again Will gave the hand signal.

"Why do you do this kind of work, Dr. Gilchrist? Dr. Rivers! Why is she taught stuff that's no damn good, that's dangerous to me?"

"Well, perhaps I overstated my case, Joe. I feel very strongly about protecting patients from bad treatment. Maybe I become too much of a crusader."

By the time the interview was over, Eve felt trashed and beaten up. To her horror, Ben had been right. He'd advised her to look for what Will was doing in addition to what he was supposed to be doing. Will was giving Joe signals that seemed to trigger abrupt changes in his attitude. Yes, Will was videotaping the interview to document his interventions and findings, but the most important aspects of the interview were off camera. The man her undergraduate professors had held up to her as a scientist's scientist first lied to her to learn about Joe, and now was undermining her efforts to help him.

How can I understand Joe's weird behavior just before the interview? If I were Ben, I would think that Will somehow got to Joe before the interview. But that still seems like some far-out conspiracy theory!

Without an aggressive word being thrown in her direction, Will had claimed the scientific high road and branded her efforts pathetic and wrong-headed. *You demeaned me, you bastard, and when you did that, you hurt Joe. You destroyed his therapy! Joe warned me if he couldn't be helped, he'd kill himself. No wonder Jordan hates you!*

NINETEEN

Ben listened to the tape. Eve said nothing about the hand signals.

"What an awful experience for you!"

"What do you mean?"

"Well, how did you feel?"

"Stupid, ashamed, wrong, beaten up … And ready to kill him."

"He put you in an impossible position, systematically undermining you and your work. I noticed some slight breaks in his tone. After each one Joe went on a tear. What else did you notice?"

"I don't want to say. It makes me feel crazy."

"That's Will. If you start to follow him down his particular road, you have to bail out, start to go crazy, or shoot him. Most people bail out. They assume that since he's smarter than the average bear, it must be that they just don't get it."

"Like Kernberg?"

"Yeah, except that Kernberg really is a genius."

"What should I think about Will?"

"He's a lying asshole. But perhaps my crude formulation is insufficiently nuanced for the cultivated Dr. Eve Gilchrist."

"Look. I feel crazy every time I start to think of saying what I'm thinking out loud."

"You want to take that home?"

"I guess not. But ... What the heck ... OK. I completely missed those subtle changes in his voice. But when those changes occurred, he was leaning to his right and holding his right arm out, with his palm flat, parallel to the ground. How crazy is that?"

"Not as crazy as not telling me."

"Look! Maybe in some alternate universe, this makes sense. But it's shaking me up too much for me to get my mind around it all."

"Bullshit, Gilchrist! Spit out the facts. Add 'em up. What do they say?"

"Really?"

"Really. Do it, or I swear I'll make you wear last year's colors."

"Well, if you want to get nasty ... Joe is a former military man who appears to have gone through some unusual training program that imposed a secondary identity upon a basic identity that remains to be clarified. Either the training was less than completely successful, a head injury destabilized that training, or something else happened to bring elements from the past and the primary identity back to the surface.

"Something powerful and/or desperate is either driving this uncovering or got unearthed by it. Two things seem to link Joe to whatever his past might have been—the importance of his high school football experience and a young lady he loved and still loves.

"He enters treatment and one of the country's most quoted psychologists jumps in for no apparent reason. He insists on intervening, and seems to have some mysterious way of communicating with Joe and manipulating his responses.

"Ergo—and God knows I don't want to say or believe it, Will Rivers probably is connected in some significant way to whatever program was training and conditioning Joe. Because he's systematically undermining any exploration of the past, I'm forced to consider that Will thinks that Joe's successful treatment would lead to the revelation of something Will doesn't want to have revealed. I don't like where this leads."

"OK. First rate!" said Ben. "Now, returning to your education. The problem isn't Will's science. He's pretending to be scientific when he's not."

"I don't get it."

"Have you ever heard the term, 'scientism'?"

"No."

"Dumbed down definition—making a show of valuing and promoting the ideas and trappings of science, whether it's appropriate for the situation or not.

"Will's scientism is a smokescreen. What he's doing is smoke and mirrors, just glib misdirections. He's focusing on memory issues.

"But putting Will's BS aside, in situations like this no matter what rock we turn over, we may get very defensive answers, if we get any at all. Parties we see as relevant sources of information may be invested in perpetuating a version of Joe Morgan's history that serves them, not Joe."

"I have to admit, I never really looked at it that carefully." Eve paused, "So, if everything is a mess, and it's hard to figure out where we could find something we can count on, where do we begin to look?"

"The answer is right in front of you. What keeps coming up for Joe Morgan, and just might escape all of these confounds?"

"I don't have the slightest idea."

"Don't underestimate yourself. You know. Let your mind drift. In empathizing, we try to walk a mile in our patients' moccasins. Trust yourself. The only thing you have to share with me is what comes up as your best guess."

Eve sat back. She closed her eyes. At first, nothing came to her. Then suddenly she found herself remembering herself as a young teen. *Whenever things were awful and I couldn't do anything about it, where would I go?*

Eve suddenly saw herself racing free as the wind, faster than any other girl on the field. Living most of her childhood abroad she grew up playing "the Beautiful Game." Football, not American football, was her outlet and escape. She saw herself back in the USA, playing soccer for a patrician girls' school, running rings around the American-raised players! She saw herself cut around one last big defender, who couldn't hold as sharp a turn. As the taller girl tripped, Eve faked to the near upper corner. The goalie committed, and Eve drilled the ball to the far lower left, barely six inches off the ground. *Goooaal!!!*

"OK, Dr. Jordan. You were right. He pretty much did tell me right off the bat. Can't you be wrong sometimes?"

"I don't like being wrong. I like teaching you to be right more often than you ever would have thought you could be."

"The dangerous thing?"

"Right. So, what did he tell you?"

Eve crumpled a sheet of paper in her right fist, and cocked her arm, "Go out for a long one, Dr. Jordan. Go deep!"

Ben caught her forward pass. "Eve! I'm so f … Scratch that. I'm so proud of you! Damn, you're good."

TWENTY

Will sat quietly, a pensive expression on his face. He nodded to Ben. Ben nodded in return. They sat in silence for a few minutes, unapologetically irritating each other.

Jeff entered breezily, shouting back over his shoulder to Sheila, "And don't disturb us. Important meeting." He seemed able to straighten his tie and his smile in a single motion.

"You two!" He shook his head. "I thought we had this all worked out."

"You did work it out, Jeff. But Ben doesn't think so."

"What's the problem, Ben?"

"The problem is that Joe Morgan's treatment with Eve Gilchrist is working toward helping him regain his identity, to recover as close to a personal history as he can get, given the vicissitudes of memory. That's what Mr. Morgan wants to achieve."

"So?"

"When Will interviewed Mr. Morgan he made a number of suggestions designed to suppress the emergence of material. That's not research. That's undermining Mr. Morgan's pursuit of his therapeutic goals."

Will sighed, shrugged to Jeff, and spoke to Ben as if he were addressing a child.

"Most knowledgeable scholars, Jeff among them, know that efforts to retrieve autobiographical memory are no better than a crapshoot. Research demonstrates that the more you push, the more you get, but what you get is likely to be nonsense, or so strongly influenced by the person pressing to get the memories out that they're likely to be confabulations that reflect the bias of the questioner."

"Ben?"

"Will is overstating his case. That research was done with word lists. Generalizing findings from word lists to complex interpersonal situations is unwarranted. Nothing supports such a wild extrapolation. Here we have an effort to go for a very different kind of material, material that, even if it's flawed, may be very helpful in giving us a place to start with this patient. It's like when hypnosis is used in certain forensic situations—you don't assume that what you find is accurate. But it may provide clues that lead to useful evidence.

"Will advocates imposing his theory-driven constraints on clinical decision-making. Those constraints have no proven worth and would reverse the direction of the therapy."

Jeff was troubled, and showed it. "Are you saying the research Will refers to is wrong, Ben? The people who did it are real heavyweights."

"Their results were solid, Ben." Will raised his voice, "My work supports them."

"There are many approaches to the subject of validity …"

"Who is the researcher here?"

"We all are, in different areas."

"With all due respect!" Will's rage exploded. "I am a scientist! You are nothing more than a pretentious wannabe who scrapes together a few observations and does an end run around weak editors and dim-witted reviewers for journals that can barely find enough garbage to fill their pages. Your papers barely limp their way over pathetically low hurdles."

Jeff cleared his throat. He looked at Will with studied diffidence.

What is going on here? Ben wondered. *Jeff never lets anyone go that far without breaking it up.*

Will continued.

"You work, Jeff, is organizational. You've set a model for the rational management of academic departments. Hell! You were cited in the *Harvard Business Review* and *Academic Psychiatry!*

"Jordan," Will pressed, "your ideas are preposterous. You want to give this man a confabulated history that never was because of your irresponsible ideas about therapy. Why? To replace a confabulated history that never was that came from God knows where? Better to help him face the truth! Whatever happened, it's gone! He has to move on! Better to help him cope with the here and now. That's good therapy. I don't know why you put up with this character. I've wasted enough time here." Will stood up and walked out of the room.

"Nice exit," Ben remarked.

"OK, Ben, what about the research angle? Does he have a point?"

"In theory, sure. Pragmatically, let's think through what follows from the strategy he suggests. 'OK, fella! For all intents and purposes your past is gone. Rather than take the risk of giving you an incomplete and possibly somewhat distorted picture of the past and continue to work to improve it and understand more and more over time, and to corroborate what we can, we recommend that you consider yourself born yesterday. If you have any loved ones who are still alive, any career you might return to, any possessions of value, any inheritance coming your way, forget about it. We won't help you try to get it back, because we might not get it completely right.' You see, it's like this, you tell the patient. 'You heard the expression half a loaf is better than none? Wrong—none of a loaf is better than half!' That leaves this man in limbo.

"Will seems comfortable with assuming god-like powers. Is it right when he claims the right to override the treatment the patient asked to have and replace it with some cock-eyed set of notions that the patient never agreed to accept? Is it right to undermine the notions that the patient did agree to accept? This falls short of malpractice only because it hasn't continued long enough to do significant damage. It's a clear dereliction of duty!

"Jeff, I'm not going to kiss your butt ..."

"That won't work, but it wouldn't hurt every now and again."

"What Will is talking about is scientism, not science. He's arguing that everything should be viewed through the lens of science as he sees it, whether or not it's relevant or accurate. His point is politically correct in a world that exists only in the minds of those so lost in their lab studies that reality has lost its meaning. And what's worse, you know he's a complete liar."

"That's a strong statement. Can you prove it?"

"Sure I can. And so can Trevor Martin and Lisa Hart and Tony Abbruzzi and Helen Bidwell. Right after the meeting we were laughing like hell. Today Will was contemptuous of basic psychodynamic psychotherapy and professed complete scorn for therapies that explore the past. But at the meeting he went on the offensive against my recommendation that we beef up our training in therapies that are actually more here and now in their focus. Now he's ranting and raving because we didn't use the kind of therapy he didn't think we needed to teach. Will says whatever serves his purpose in the moment and calls it science."

"OK. OK. That last point is a good one. I missed it the first time around. But it changes nothing."

"While you're thinking of changing nothing consider this. Nothing Will said has ecological validity. Remember ecological validity? The notion that it's important to demonstrate that what you can prove under some circumstances also holds under other circumstances before you decide it's a general truth? That's important."

"Yeah. You do have a point. OK, OK. He completely blindsided me there, too. You're right. Here's the bottom-line: He made his point. You made yours. I'll make mine. Will can continue his research with Joe Morgan. You don't have to like it."

"I don't. When you look back on it, you won't either."

"I can live with that."

TWENTY-ONE

Eve sat red-faced and speechless. Her usual composure had vanished. She always pushed herself to excel, and was unaccustomed to failure. Her session with Joe Morgan had been soul shattering. She could barely push through her mortification.

Ben watched Eve place the tape on his player, and waited for her to speak. She said nothing. Finally, she forced herself to play the tape.

Joe launched one irrational, vicious attack after another against Eve. She said nothing as the insults kept coming. Ben stopped the tape.

"Eve, I'm getting worried. You're really taking a licking in this session. What's going on?"

Still nothing.

"I'll wait."

Finally, Eve spoke.

"I must have done something very wrong." Her eyes filled with tears. "I'm so sorry."

"Rather than jump to conclusions, let's listen carefully to what it is that you're talking about."

Eve nodded and wiped away her tears. *Classic Ben Jordan. Nothing warm and fuzzy, just ruthless problem solving*. The tape continued. Joe Morgan went after Eve with venomous hatred, challenging virtually every observation she made. Then he began to ask her who she really was. Sometimes he stopped, expressed confusion, and went on a tirade again.

Joe Morgan sounded acutely psychotic, as if he had developed paranoid irrational negative beliefs and misgivings about Eve in just a matter of days. Ben was sure that "the Universal Attractor" was pretty much a rookie at being disliked. More and more, Ben appreciated Jeff's wisdom in treating Eve so protectively, in bringing her along so slowly and gently. Therapists must learn to tolerate, contain, and work with irrational negative accusations that their patients may believe are accurate descriptions of the therapist's shortcomings, but usually reflect bad experiences and disappointments from the past, sometimes linked to issues in the here and now.

"This mess is being dumped on you, Eve, but you didn't cause it. We've had indications Joe can have problems with reality testing under stress. That's not unusual in high hypnotizables, dissociatives, whatever … It seems logical to assume there could be some intervening variable that might have messed things up. If we wonder along that line, what are our best suspects?"

Eve rallied, and began to pull herself out of her funk.

"Some post-traumatic trigger, probably beneath the level of his awareness, kind of like Arthur Blank just wrote about—unconscious flashbacks to an earlier trauma. An intercurrent medical illness that affects the central nervous system—traumatic, infectious, inflammatory, seizure-like or seizure-related, maybe related to a developing tumor or neurological condition. A reaction to a drug or other chemical. Or … and I hate to say this—some unfortunate psychosocial influence."

"Like Willie and his hand jive. Good. Let's listen to some more."

No matter how many ways you change, I know who you are. I don't know why you try to tell me you are my doctor. Well maybe you're my doctor, too. The timing fits. You had just enough time to go to college and medical school and be a resident. I thought you loved me. I thought you would wait for me. But you must have married someone rich, with all the rings and gold. I guess I wasn't good enough for you. Just a Marine. You broke my heart, damn you! I ought to kill you.

Joe! I'm confused. Do you think you're mixing me up with a girl you loved? A girl you may have known when things were very different? You've told me that you've called a girl you were dating by a different name.

"At this point, I saw Joe's eyes began to close. He put his hands to his temples, like for a bad headache."

Eve let the tape continue.

Ah! This pain is awful!

Sometimes when you talk about the things you are studying, you can come back to the here and now. How are your classes going?

I don't think I can talk about that! I'm not sure who you are right now. Oh, my God! Why did you cut your hair? Who gave you all those gold things?

This has got to be confusing, and maybe frightening and enraging. That headache tells us that whatever is going on in your mind is causing a lot of conflict. It seems that there may have been a girl in your past that was very important to you, and that when you look at me, sometimes you see her instead of me, or images of her and images of me switch back and forth.

Yeah! Why do you do that?

Actually, Joe, I wish to God I knew why this is happening and how to get it straightened out for you.

You could! You could! That scientist guy said all sorts of things about what you're doing wrong! I can't trust you any more. You're some kind of fraud! Why aren't you doing what that big shot said you should do?

Eve stopped the tape.

"I've never faced anything like this. Joe seemed genuinely unsure about who I was. It was one thing to hear you preaching doom and gloom if Will undermined my work with Joe, but this is all too real! Joe looked like he was going to attack me. This is much, much too real! He scared me. I guess I didn't really believe you. I mean I guess I did, but I guess at a deeper level I really didn't. You thought that confronting Joe with contradictory treatment approaches would create a dangerous situation. I must have been feeling, 'Yeah. Yeah. But that can't happen here!'

"Now I get what 'double bind' really means. Joe is trying to make sense of the chaos this double bind creates, and he's coming up with paranoid theories to make some sense of it all. To Joe, I'm the doctor in charge. He's accusing me of making things go wrong."

Ben nodded, and said, "Before we talk about the double bind, remember that Will planted some pretty strong suggestions that you're a dangerous person doing dangerous treatment. I can't overemphasize how toxic that is.

"The essence of a double bind involves three main factors. First, there has to be a primary injunction. Here that would be the chosen direction of treatment—'Work to recover and understand your past as well as possible.' Then there's a second injunction contradicting the first. Here, that would come from the suggestions Will and others put into the mix and go like this: 'You can't recover your past, and anything you might seem to recover is probably an illusion that might deceive you in very significant ways. Anyone who tries to tell you or treat you otherwise is dangerous to your mental health.'"

"Will and others?"

"Allow me my paranoia. No proof, just suspicions. Third, the person caught between the first two injunctions can't get away, can't abandon the field. That's the formula for being driven more than a bit crazy. You're being messed with and you really can't get away. Even if it's physically possible, it may not be psychologically possible. We have to understand how the way Joe is acting, however horrible and distressing it is to you and to him, may represent his best effort to escape the double bind and strike back against what's driving him crazy. According to Will, that's you. He goes crazy one way in the belief that what he's doing protects him from being driven crazy in another way.

"Let's hear some more. I don't imagine it's going to be pretty."

"That's for sure," Eve sighed.

> *You're not a real doctor. You pretend to be my doctor and you go and fuck me up.*

Eve stopped the tape at once. "Joe got out of his chair. He paced around for a few seconds, but in that linen closet-sized office of mine, there's nowhere to go. Then he got up in my face. He leaned over me, shouting and shaking his fist in my face, kind of spitting in my face."

"I'm sorry, Eve. You don't deserve that."

The tape resumed.

> *Now I know you're all frauds! Everyone who pretends to care—my family, my friends, my teachers, my coaches—you're all fakes! I don't know how you all learned how to act like the real people in my life, but the real people are lost! All of you, you*

fuckin' fakers, you're such fuckin' pieces of shit to be doing this to me! I should get the hell out of here and do every one of you!

One loud crash was followed by another, and then by a deafening slam.

"That," Eve told Ben Jordan, "was the chart being torn out of my hands and thrown against the wall, the tape recorder being thrown on the floor and shattering into a million pieces, and my composure being blasted into oblivion as Joe Morgan exited, stage left, slamming the door so hard that he literally tore it off one of its hinges."

"I'm so sorry, Eve. This is the kind of crap I was afraid Will's bullshit would cause. I know you're giving yourself all sorts of grief. Give yourself a break. The best player can't beat a stacked deck."

"But I don't get it. What on earth is happening?"

"Apart from Will's setting you up to get your face smashed? Apart from his setting it up so he can run to Jeff and say, 'I warned you! Save the department from disaster and disgrace!' Apart from that and all the other sinister somethings that would make all of this make sense? Not much.

"Now, putting aside Will's disgusting behavior for the moment, have you ever heard of conditions in which people come to believe that important people in their lives aren't real—that they've been replaced by doubles, by identical impostors?"

"Uh—isn't it that syndrome that sounds like 'crabgrass'?"

Ben laughed. "Yeah. Capgras syndrome. Get it straight before you take your specialty boards. What about a syndrome in which your enemies or people you know can take on the appearance of strangers? The person begins to think that different people are in fact the same person who changes appearance or who appears to be in disguise."

"Will they ask that on the boards?"

"Who knows?"

"My mind is blank."

"The Fregoli syndrome."

"I'm lost."

"OK. Let's think this through together. Both syndromes usually occur with schizophrenia or seizure activities. Our boy is not schizophrenic. All bets are off about organic problems, including seizures. But here's an interesting wrinkle.

"Directed misperceptions are common challenges in hypnosis research. In one major scale, you suggest away knowledge of a particular number, and watch the subject make up, confabulate ways to get around it. In Orne's double hallucination test, you convince a person to have a hallucination of your assistant, whom they've met, while that person is out of the room. And then you have the assistant come back, and now the subject sees two images of your assistant. Stage hypnotists have similar tricks.

"But let's put ourselves in the position of someone who is diabolically clever, who may have trained someone to hallucinate a particular face on another person and react to that other person as if they were the person whose face they see. Consider creating iatrogenic Capgras and Fregoli symptoms in order to manipulate someone."

"How would someone do that?"

"Rehearsals, misdirection."

"I'm lost. Why?"

"OK. Suppose I want to prepare you to assassinate the president."

"Thanks."

"I can tell you to shoot the president all day, but will you do it? If I've conditioned you to believe in the reality of switched faces, I might instruct you to see one person as another."

"My God!"

"Suppose I train you so that the moment you see the president under certain circumstances, you will perceive him as a notorious international terrorist who must be there to kill the president. Ergo, being a patriotic American, you blow that no-good bastard to pieces to save the president."

"I don't like what I'm hearing!"

"Can't say I blame you. So. If this guy is having flashbacks of an old girlfriend and they're afraid his love for her will overcome his conditioning, they might …"

"Convince him that the real girlfriend is dead or gone, or no darn good, and whoever he might think is her is really someone else who is no good at all, maybe even an enemy. Confuse him so that every time he sees me, he confuses me with her because on and off I seem to have her face, and now I'm no damn good either. It's just a hop, skip, and jump into sending him off to actually eliminate the people whom he cares about, and who might break the hold of his training. My God! Do you think he might kill me?"

"Possibly. But the people at the top of something like this probably understand that killing the daughter of a prominent political figure might trigger problems they'd like to avoid. If my paranoid construction of things is on target, that would be their last resort. I think Plan A is to frighten you away and discredit my efforts, extricating Joe from our influence. If they're scared enough about you and me, whoever is handling Joe may decide it's best all around to go to Plan B, take him down so he never can spill the beans. Of course that leaves us as loose ends. Perhaps Plan C, then it might come down to 'Psychotic ex-Marine slaughters young psychiatrist and middle-aged professor.' We're in a high-risk profession."

Ben sat for a moment.

"OK. I have a plan to get around all of this and track down the truth. You guessed the starting point. It's an idea I have to explore—alone."

"Why?"

"Forces have been exerted to get Joe bent out of shape, and the way he's getting bent out of shape endangers you. At a very important level all that matters is that you could get hurt. That's just not acceptable."

"Hippocrates?"

"Hippocrates' maxim even applies to lower forms of life like residents. I have to take you off the case."

"No!"

"Not negotiable!"

"But ..."

"Not negotiable! This is a very volatile situation. It may be beyond my skill set, too, but it's my job to deal with the very difficult stuff. It's your job to build up your skills and experience and become a go-to person down the road."

"How about co-therapy?"

"I thought of that, but if he's really in the grip of some psychotic misperceptions of you and crazy commands to act on those misperceptions, I think you get the picture. Maybe I can tape him and we'll learn together. I feel lousy about taking you off the case, but I'd feel a hell of a lot worse if something happened to hurt you, physically, psychologically, or career-wise."

"Is that your final offer?"

"Yes. If you were my kid, I'd pull you out. I can't do any less for you. Now, let me think about loose ends. Have you heard from BI in Boston?"

"Not yet."

"Well, before I throw you out of something I think is bad, maybe I can do one simple thing that could give you more insight into just how convoluted this whole thing may be."

"How do you mean?"

"I remember the general telephone number for Beth Israel in Boston. I had a few rotations there as a medical student."

An operator connected Ben to Medical Records at BI.

"This is Professor Jordan at the U in Philadelphia. I'm calling in follow-up of a request for medical records on a Joe Morgan ... Lots of luck? Hah! That hasn't changed since I was there a million years ago … Yeah, really! Internal medicine and psych. No, it's not an emergency. And don't tell me I still have old charts to sign! All I really need to know today is that you got our request. Our Dr. Gilchrist sent it in."

Ben turned to Eve.

"They're transferring me to a supervisor … Hmm. That couldn't be him. Our Joe Morgan is a young guy, D.O.B. 11/2/58 is on the chart. Can you look by date of birth and see if there is any youngish guy who had a bunch of CNS studies late last year, or earlier this year? Nada. Zilch. Thanks anyway. Any chance you could transfer me to the office of Mantosh Chadawarry in neurology? Thanks."

Ben turned to Eve. "The name of the neurologist Joe said he saw is probably real, though he didn't get it right. I had to present a case to him when I was a student."

"How did that go?"

"About as well as when you first presented Joe to me. Shit! She's telling him who's calling. Shit! Shit! Shit!"

Eve pressed the speakerphone button.

"For that, you will die a slow death!"

Eve stuck out her tongue, put her thumbs in her ears, and wiggled her fingers.

"Ah, Dr. Jordan!" Eve enjoyed watching the sound of Chadawarry's smooth, Indian accent induce rising panic in her usually calm and collected consultant. "Always good to hear from an old student and friend! How can I help you?"

"Well, sir, I have a signed release of information paper from a man who may be our mutual patient, but I'm not sure that he actually came to see you. You needn't trouble yourself, sir. Your secretary can answer that particular question."

"Sir?" whispered Eve.

"Ah, old wounds, Ben Jordan! Old wounds! We must move on, old fellow. Vi? I will give you a name."

Ben provided the name and date of birth for the man Eve was seeing.

"Vi, was he seen in our office, by me, earlier this year?"

There was laughter from several female voices in the background.

"No," said Chadawarry. He lost his composure and began to laugh.

"Dr. Jordan. Do you know why we are all laughing, every single one of us?"

"No. Will I respect myself in the morning?"

"I doubt it … OK, I owe you a straight answer even though it has been fun to relive old times. Remember that fateful day?"

"No. Every time I come near remembering it, I beat my head against concrete for an hour."

"You must remember in order to learn! I recall that you presented a case with eloquence and brilliance, but there were some problems with the facts?"

"Through the dim mists."

"You did it again!"

"I get it! I should have asked whether you were even around then."

"Correct! Too little, too late, but finally correct! I was doing research at the Karolinska Institute with Tor Svensson. I just got back. Ben, you are brilliant—sometimes. But first you have to plod along with the rest of us and get your facts straight. Vi! While I was away, did anyone else in our department see a man with the name or the nature of problems our old student is concerned about? No? Nothing, Ben. Sorry I can't help you."

Ben stared at the wall.

"After all these years, he remembers you and teases you?"

"It's a long story."

"Something that would help a resident understand the great ones?"

"Good try, Eve. No, but it may help you learn about traumatic triggers. I was so rattled when Chadawarry got on the line that I went into that old emotional stuff and didn't remember to ask him what every rookie cop learns to ask. You just witnessed a cognitive regression."

"So if you were more with it today, it would have been a 'Where were you on the night of June 21st?' kind of thing."

"Yep. If Joe has no records at BI and hot shot Chadawarry was overdosing on saunas, reindeer steaks, and cloudberries instead of testing Joe's reflexes, what the hell happened to make a young army reservist, who's supposed to have been hit by a tank and suffered head trauma become somewhat disoriented to the present, become flooded with images that suggest that some unknown past is popping into his awareness, and become able to give a detailed description of a work-up at a Harvard teaching hospital that never occurred, including offering a convincing description of his encounter with a medical luminary that he's never met?

"Put this together with the other stuff, the misperceptions, and it's not too far-fetched to figure that someone is actively monkeying with Joe Morgan's mind. That's pretty high-powered stuff!

"I really wish we could continue to work on this together. You've demonstrated an astonishing capacity to grow, and to grow very rapidly. Since the medical records are a dead end, now it's time for football. Tell Jeff I'll fill him in personally, but that you're off the case because Joe's developed a psychotic negative transference, torn up your office, and threatened to kill you. Tell him that I don't think that this is a case that any resident can treat safely. Don't share my suspicions about Will. That's going to be a bad scene. Keep out of it."

TWENTY-TWO

"In essence, Dr. Jordan said, 'Come back in ten or fifteen years and you may be ready for Joe Morgan. I'm not sure I'm ready for him myself.'"

Jeff was silent for a moment. Then he smiled sadly.

"He's right. Hell, I'm not ready for Joe Morgan. Ben has a unique skill set. And he's been there. And … There's a lot of ands. I hope you get a chance to work with him again on a case that's not full of land mines and quicksand. He has a lot to teach. I'm sorry about this whole mess.

"I'm glad to see you're out of it. Will was really pushing to protect you from this situation. I'm glad Ben came around to the same point of view."

Jeff is distorting the facts to make Will look good! It reminded Eve of how her father approached certain diplomatic situations, struggling to make them win-win, or at least to make them appear win-win.

* * *

After Eve left his office, Jeff poured himself some Highland Park. Living a lie was wreaking havoc with his conscience.

On her way out of the department's office suites, Eve encountered Lisa Hart. When she saw the concern in Lisa's kind eyes, she almost lost control. She dashed off before Lisa had a chance to reach out to her.

Her chest tightened. The tears came, bitter and unwanted. Eve had trusted Jeff since medical school. She had idealized Will Rivers since her first year of college. Now both had lied and betrayed her. Eve suddenly felt much younger, a little girl helpless and alone, engulfed by despair.

TWENTY-THREE

Eve prayed she could reach her office unnoticed, but Bobby Gray looked up and called to her as she passed his open door.

"Eve!"

"Hi, Bobby!"

"Could you come in for a second?"

Eve slumped down in a chair. Bobby closed the door.

"I'm worried. This is the first time I've ever seen you look—well, like shit. Are you OK?"

"I'm OK, Bobby. Just ..."

"Just? Just what?"

"I don't want to talk about it."

"Well, you sure don't look like a happy camper. Knowing you, I doubt you're in any personal therapy. Where are you going to go with this?"

Eve cursed the tear escaping down her cheek.

"Look. I don't like spreading my private business all over the place."

"Granted. But if you walk around like this, you won't have to spread your secrets. They're going to scream, 'Here we are!'"

"Yeah. I think Lisa made me on the way over."

"She's sharp. And sweet."

Eve chuckled. "Yeah, I get the hint. I guess I'm one of those 'therapy is for those other people' kind of shrinks."

"Yeah. That's where I started. Changed my mind."

"Did that get held against you?"

"No. At first I only told Jordan. But Jeff is much sharper than he likes to show. He noticed some changes and said, 'Whatever you're doing that's different, keep on doing it.' He knew. I don't make a secret of it."

"I'm not in that kind of trouble. But I could use your advice."

"Mine?"

"Yeah. I'm trying to avoid taking a hit when the big dogs go after one another."

"Which big dogs? Over which bone?"

Eve chuckled, "There's this case …"

"Oh, shit! The one with memory and identity problems?"

"How did you know?"

"It came up indirectly at the departmental meeting. Ben was advocating for more training in some modalities. Jeff backed him, and mentioned a case example to show why Ben was right. Don't worry. Jeff was ferocious about preserving confidentiality. He just said that a gifted resident was treating the person. There was a back and forth involving the usual suspects, plus Will Rivers, who was particularly nosy. So, in view of Jeff's high opinion of you, and your exuberant expression, I guess you're the one in the middle of this mess."

"Yeah. Ben wants to figure things out as much as possible, but Will's on some crusade I don't understand. He's discouraging that approach and getting really steamed at Ben. I've learned so darn much—I want to see this through.

"But Ben just threw me off the case. Well, the patient trashed my office and threatened me. Ben said he wouldn't allow me to get caught in some silly battle that could hurt my career, or to continue some treatment that might get me hurt.

"I don't know … Will is supposed to be this super-scholar. I had to read his papers in college. My psychology profs thought he was a god. Jeff has been a wonderful mentor. And Ben is—very different, almost ferocious in what he does. He has a lot to offer. But they're into some idiotic squabble. Don't you think this good shrink/bad shrink stuff is all too dramatic?"

Bobby sat silent long enough for Eve to wonder if he had drifted off.

"Bobby? What do you think?"

"Eve, I don't have your magical way of saying things just right so everyone is happy and no one feels bruised. If you repeat what I'm about to say, I'll deny that I said it. Got it?"

"I'm surprised, but I got it."

"Jeff is a very good man, but when push comes to shove, he's a politician. Ben is a very good man, but when push comes to shove, he's a warrior. Both will do everything they can to do the right thing, but every now and then they have different ideas of what's right. Push comes to shove, Jeff will do what's he thinks is best for the department, plus/minus for Jeff. Push comes to shove, Ben will do what is best for whomever he cares about. He may get around to worrying about the other stuff later."

"Bobby? You didn't say anything about Will."

"Uh, yeah."

"Bobby?"

"If Ben says steer clear, steer clear."

"Bobby, Will is supposed to be some research genius. He and Ben are at odds, and Jeff seems to be backing Will. Help me make sense of this."

Bobby again went silent. Finally, he spoke.

"I'm breaking a million rules in telling you this. But in my heart, I feel it's the right thing to do. I don't like doing this, but I don't want to see you get screwed."

Bobby was silent another minute.

"Once, when Ben was overseas with his National Guard unit, there was a crisis with one of his patients. Whoever was covering couldn't be reached. I was on call. Jeff asked me to handle it.

"This young woman was sun bathing on a beach down in Delaware. She suddenly noticed a man was looking at her, you know, the way guys can look. It freaked her out."

"That sounds hysterical."

"That's what I thought. But she was a faculty member's patient, so what could I do? I saw her. Bottom line, the problem was who was staring at her. It was a mental health professional she claimed had molested her."

"That's awful."

"Worse still. It was Dr. Brewer, Will's buddy. She was at the U. She went to Student Health and complained."

Eve played dumb.

"Ben Jordan?"

"Yep. She said Ben reported Brewer, but Will stepped in and bamboozled Darymple and her parents. She tried to kill herself. When she needed help and had no money or insurance, Ben saw her pro bono, under an alias. She was doing great … until she saw Brewer."

"What did you do?"

"What had to be done. I can't say I didn't shit a brick until Jordan got back. He was ready to explode when he found out I'd been dragged into this, but he calmed down. Well, after he smashed something. Then he apologized to me for the situation and his outburst, and got on the phone to his patient."

"So?"

"Trust Jordan first, Jeff second, and never trust Will or Brewer. If Jordan pulled you off, it's because he's protective. He's doing what he thinks he needs to do."

TWENTY-FOUR

Ben couldn't reach Joe Morgan, but his roommate answered.

"Joe's out of town. He said he was visiting some girl."

He promised to pass along Ben's message. To cover himself and the U, Ben followed up with a certified letter, offering Joe treatment by a senior psychiatrist, still covered by his insurance. He asked Joe to call to arrange an appointment.

TWENTY-FIVE

Joe Morgan remembered attending Somerset High School. Ben learned there was no "Somerset High" during Joe's teens. Kids in Somerset generally went to Somerset Berkeley Regional High School, or crossed the Taunton River to Bishop Connolly, a Catholic high school in nearby Fall River.

The school secretary fielded his call. He learned that most locals called the regional school "Somerset High" anyway. The distinction was trivial and picky, but Ben wondered why a man trying to find himself and validate his memories of his past hadn't given Eve the school's full name. *Does that mean something, or am I just being obsessive?*

Ben was transferred to the principal, Dr. Paul Reimer. Reimer bombarded him with hard questions, offering nothing until his suspicions were allayed.

"So … you need my assistance to help a patient?"

"Not just any patient. He's a guy who says he's from Massachusetts, and he sounds that way."

Reimer laughed, "The kind who paahks his caah in Haaahvahd Yaahd?"

"No, the kind that has 'idears'." Ben was stretching, but he hoped the detail would amuse Reimer. Often Boston drops 'r's, southern Mass adds them.

"That's more my neck of the woods."

"He was on active duty with his National Guard unit. He suffered a head injury and was unconscious for a while. He was mixed up about his life even before that. He insists that he graduated from your school and played football there some year you were state champs, but ..."

"Is this the guy who tried to find his old coach a while back?"

"The same."

"Poor bastard! I still put in my weekend and screw up my summers."

"Yeah, me too. New Jersey Air."

"OK. What can I do to help you help this guy? He could be me ... or you, for that matter."

"That's for sure. Two things. First, if I fax you his picture, can someone check it against the yearbook pictures and team pictures for a couple years?"

"No problem. I'll do that myself tonight. I've been at this school as a student, teacher, assistant principal ... Except for college, grad school, and 'Nam, forever. I should be able to get that done."

"Second thing ... Could you connect me with your football coach? I have a few questions I need to ask him."

"Look, I want to help, but I can't OK him saying anything about any student."

"Glad to hear you say that. No, I want to ask him about his team's schedule and opponents for a period of years."

"That's odd."

"I'm a shrink. I do odd."

"Let me warn you, Bill Buchholz, our football coach, thinks psychiatry is a bunch of bullshit. But for someone who served, he'll give you the shirt off his back. Let me call first."

TWENTY-SIX

"Hello, this is the Buchholz residence." The voice on the telephone was bright and airy, the happy melody of a teenage girl full of life.

"I don't suppose that you're Coach Buchholz?"

"Not likely! Dad! It's for you!"

"Hello. This is Bill Buchholz." The voice was deep, mild and calm.

"I'm Ben Jordan …"

"The shrink?"

"Yes."

"I don't care much for shrinks or the pussies that go to them."

Ben heard "Dad!" from the coach's daughter. He could just see her rolling her eyes.

"I guess that bit's a real crowd-pleaser."

Ben heard a soft chuckle.

"OK. Reimer told me to expect your call. He's the boss."

"Some days the chain of command can be a real bitch."

"Ain't that the truth? What can I do for you?"

"First, if you hear me out and want me to take a long walk on a short pier, that's your call. Here's the situation.

"I'm consulting on a guy who suffered some trauma, probably head trauma, while serving in the National Guard. He looks OK on the outside, but inside he's a complete mess. It's like he forgot who he was, like he patched together some identity that worked for a while, but now it's falling apart. The way he talks, he did a couple hitches in the Marines, got out, and went to college. But he's lost most of his past. He's running around trying to figure out who he really is. He's misperceiving people and beginning to get pretty aggressive. He got pretty belligerent with his doctor, a young woman. Somehow, he has a lot of stuff in his head that may be memories, may be God knows what. But I'm trying to help his doctor help him ..."

"So why am I talking to you instead of his doctor?"

"The resident doctor who was working with him has no experience at all with this kind of situation, and things have gotten dangerous. I have some background knowledge of how minds get messed up this way. I just took over the case in the last 24 hours."

"Brainwashing stuff?

"Yeah."

"Where did you learn that?"

"Can't tell you in any detail. You probably can't tell me why that jumped right to the top of your list."

Buchholz chuckled.

"But I can say that I am currently a colonel in the New Jersey Air Force National Guard, and served with the Israeli Defense Forces in another lifetime."

"As a doctor?

"No."

There was a long silence.

"You met this guy."

"Yeah. Poor bastard. You blew your bullshit head trauma story."

"That was the straw that broke the camel's back, not the main event. It's my icebreaker when I talk to people who think I'm a witch doctor and that everyone who comes to me is a pussy. Starting off that way may seem like bullshit to you, but we docs call it the chief complaint and presenting symptoms, basically his ticket of admission into treatment. Sorry if you thought I was jerking you around. Starting with what brings the patient to us is just an old witch doctor trick."

"OK." The coach's voice was softer now. "What do you want?"

"I want to know your opponents in football for certain years. I want to get copies of your schedule those years. I want to know the colors of their uniforms, and their team nicknames."

"What the hell? Hey! You are a clever SOB! I see what you're up to."

"I hope not. They'll take away my chicken bones and rattles. But one more thing … He was talking about a Coach MacDonald."

"Yeah. He never coached here."

"Do you know of any coach with that name?"

"Not around here. You know, if he was into sports, he could have had dozens of coaches, from Little League and Peewee Football on. I don't know any way to check all of those possibilities. Ready to take some notes?"

"Sure."

* * *

Buchholz was brisk and efficient. Within minutes Ben had the information he needed about high school football in southern Massachusetts.

A few minutes later Dr. Reimer called.

"Was Bill civil?"

"Just like you called it. He's sneaky smart."

"He came here as a physics teacher, would you believe? Stepped in as coach midseason when the guy before him had a heart attack. But, back to your guy. I checked his name and picture against the years you mentioned, and for five years before and after."

"Was that for extra credit?"

"Yeah, right. Sorry. I couldn't find anyone who resembled him. If you have more pictures, I'll look again."

TWENTY-SEVEN

Ben sat quietly as Jeff paced back and forth, blowing off steam. A member of the U's board of directors had just read him the riot act, and he was shaken.

"This guy's the CFO of a Fortune 500 company. He didn't know what he was talking about, but that didn't seem to matter. He was irate with me for allowing things to get out of control and endanger major funding streams."

"Allowing? Streams?"

"Oh, crap! Forget I said that." Jeff and Ben locked eyes. "Fat chance, eh?"

Ben smiled sadly.

"So what we know about is only one arm of the octopus?"

"I didn't say this. But … You bet!"

"Sorry, Jeff. That means that big bucks pour into the U from sources that are fastidiously disguised …"

"Don't go there, Ben!"

"We wake up in a pile of pig shit up to our necks and receive a direct order to smell sweet? What do you want to bet that this CFO big shot has ties to Glenville-Rogers? Should I check out their board of directors?"

"Has anyone told you recently that really smart people can be colossal pains in the ass?"

"If it comes to that, put some gin in my hemlock."

"You're not that smart."

Sheila apologized for intruding. "I'm sorry, Jeff. The operator just transferred a call for Ben over here. It could be important. A Mr. Buchholz?"

"Excuse me, Jeff. This regards the case that lights up your heart."

"Getting anywhere? Please say 'No!'"

* * *

Ben found a quiet place to take the call.

"Coach? Ben Jordan."

"OK. This may not mean anything. But just on the chance it might help that poor bastard, here it is. My son goes to UMass. He and his roommate were here last weekend. They were bitching about their line coach. He's busting their balls about off-season conditioning. I mean, I listened, but their coach is right. No sarcasm, Dr. Jordan."

"I'll save it for another time."

"Appreciated. In any case, I was talking to his roommate while my son went out to pick up some pizzas. Pizzas! I'm like Rodney Dangerfield in my own house! But it seems this fella played his high school ball in Nantucket."

"The Whalers!"

"Right. Just like New Bedford, but their colors are blue and white, by the way. So he was talking about how much he respected his high school coach, Mike Fletcher. I know Mike, but not well. He's an absolutely great guy. So this kid goes on bitch, moan, and groaning and then he says, 'I wish I was still playing for Coach Mack.'"

"Coach Mack?"

"Yeah. Jordan, sometimes I think folks like you and me must take stupid pills so we don't see shit that's right in front of our eyes."

"I'm still overdosed. What are you saying?"

"Jordan—MacDonald is this guy's first name. He calls himself Mike, but his name is MacDonald Fletcher. The kids call him Mr. Mack. From what your guy says about his coach, and what my kid's roommate says, and what I know, this is the kind of guy you'll want to check out. His players love him. He's the kind of guy that really goes the extra yard for every kid on his team. His house is always open to them. He's the kind of coach …"

"That resembles you?"

"On a good day. I wish. He's a coach's coach."

"Coach?"

"Yeah?"

"If you have figured out what I'm up to, please keep it to yourself. You're way smarter than the average bear, and I may have only one shot at breaking through."

"Understood. If someone really did mess with that kid, you're talking about big dogs. Just one thing?"

"Name it."

"If this isn't all bullshit, and if there really is some bastard who messed up that kid, and if you catch that bastard?"

"Yeah?"

"Send him to Somerset. We broke a tackling dummy last year, and the board was too cheap to replace it."

Ben hung up and returned to Jeff's office.

"That coach is dangerously intelligent. I think he gave me the key to that patient's past."

"Be careful what you wish for, Ben. I'm still concerned that this could be a wild goose chase."

"Of course it could. But unlike the true geniuses over in the research building, I don't know in advance whether something is right or wrong. I'm one of those backwoods types that gets serious about the difference between proof and speculation."

"Are you sure you're not just an arrogant asshole who's going to fuck things up beyond redemption?"

"Even if you don't give a shit about what's really happening under your nose, try to give a shit about Eve Gilchrist. Ask her to play you that last tape, and you tell me if you want her anywhere near this case.

"And by the way, I discussed Joe's case with the neurologist in Boston who saw him."

"Yeah?"

"He never was there."

TWENTY-EIGHT

Joe made no response to Ben's efforts to reach him. Ben decided to make a house call.

Joe and his roommate Marty Franks lived in a garden apartment on the outskirts of the city. *This place reeks of money!* The cars in the parking areas were distinctly upscale. *Not a Beetle in the bunch!* The women he saw chatting and walking their dogs were dressed to impress. *They're wearing Elani!* His wife's apparel line was upscale and costly. *Why are two undergrads just out of the service living in a place that's got to be absurdly expensive and so damn far from campus?*

Ben simply knocked on the door and took his chances. A muscular young man about six foot two answered.

"Marty Franks," he stuck out his hand, and helped Ben appreciate the power of his grip.

"I'm sorry," said Franks, mouthing the disingenuous apology of men who enjoy intimidating others. "I work out."

"Really? Nothing wrong with that."

"What can I do for you?"

"I'm Dr. Jordan from Student Health at the U. Joe came in and we've sort of lost track of him, so I dropped by to see if I could invite him to drop in and say hello."

"Why did Joe go to Student Health?"

"That I can't say. Confidentiality. I'm sure you understand."

"Sure. Sure." Marty was in a bind. Even with the reconditioning sessions, Joe was continuing to slip away. *If I hurry him out, he may get suspicious. Let me get some sense of this guy. Someday I'll probably have to kill him.*

Franks was surprised that his crushing grip had made no impact. *Was Jordan slapping me back with that "Really?"*

"Well, darn if I know where he is. Joe could be anywhere. Come on in. Let me see if he left some message somewhere. I haven't been a good friend to Joe the last few days. I messed up in one course. My prof gave me an extra week to get it right this time. I just don't want to screw up again and wind up with an incomplete, you know?"

"Sure. You don't need that hanging over you."

"No I don't. I'm just not a natural student. But, you need the sheepskin to get ahead. Right?"

Ben walked into the apartment.

"It's probably been a long time since you lived like this, Dr. Jordan."

"To tell you the truth, you guys are neat freaks compared to my college roommates."

"Give me a minute." Marty opened a cold Coke for Ben without asking if he wanted one, and disappeared into another room. Ben sat and waited.

"Sorry. I can't find anything."

"Well, thanks for your hospitality. I left my card near that pile of mail over there. Whenever Joe shows up, please tell him to give me a call."

"You got it. Nice to meet you, sir."

Marty saw Ben out. Then he sat down and began to write a memorandum about Jordan's unexpected visit.

Ben Jordan lingered a few moments in his car. He thought he saw a figure crouching in the shadows of the shrubs surrounding the next building over. He considered either waiting or leaving and rapidly returning with his lights out. Neither alternative seemed helpful.

After Ben drove off, Joe entered the apartment.

"Who was our visitor?"

Marty pointed to the card.

"Your mystery caller and pen-pal. Dr. Jordan. That's his card. I thought you said your doctor was this really good-looking woman."

"Yeah. This guy must have been her supervisor. I don't remember much of my last session. Maybe—maybe something went wrong. I guess he's a big shot, and they want some big shot to take over."

"Well, if big shot means more experience, more knowledge, that might be good if what's bugging you is too much for a beginner to handle."

"I don't know, Marty. I just hate walking around feeling that I'm so fucked up. Fucked up enough to need a shrink, and fucked up enough to need some super-shrink? I haven't felt right since my folks died. That really messed me up."

"Well, I see you every day. Now, maybe I'm a dope, but most of the time you seem pretty normal to me, pal. Whatever it is, get it fixed. You deserve to get it together. Look. I'm no shrink. I wish I knew what to tell you. But I don't, and I'm wasted. I've got to crash."

"Just one thing, Marty. What sort of guy was this Jordan?"

"Who knows? Seemed friendly enough. We just talked for a couple of minutes. Didn't say much except about locating you and asking you to come in. He's around six foot—a couple inches shorter than me. Maybe 180. Dark hair, big smile. Pretty solid. Looks like a guy who stays in great shape. Lots of scars on his hands. He must have a story."

"I'll call him and get him off my back. Yours too. Good night."

* * *

An hour later, Marty Franks placed a call. He hung up after four rings. Minutes later he called again and Will answered on the fourth ring.

"Marty?" *It has to be something big to call at this hour.*

"What a mess! Some of those tests didn't turn out so great. Nick's going to need some serious treatment."

"Oh, shit! I'm sorry to hear that."

"He's taken some time off. I'm going to drop in and say hello as soon as I can."

"I will, too. Maybe I'll bring along another old friend of his. Thanks for calling."

They would have to talk in person. Will left a message at his office to clear the time the following morning. Then he called a number Joe's Ares state would answer. When a sleepy voice answered, Will said,

"N, A, M, S. Reunion. 4. Record."

Had Johnson left the message, it would say,

"Nick, Ares, Mars, and Seth. Come back to the lab at 4 p.m. tomorrow. Write down the appointment."

TWENTY-NINE

Ben reached MacDonald Fletcher, Coach Mack, early the following afternoon.

"I'm a psychiatrist in Philadelphia. I'm working with a patient who lost his memory, or had his memory tampered with."

"How does this connect to me?"

"It may not. But if there's something that links you to him, a few minutes of your time may save this guy's sanity. Maybe his life."

"OK, but I have a house full of people here. Maybe we should talk later."

"Three minutes max. I promise."

"Shoot."

"He says he played for a Coach Mack. Remember the championship year for the Whalers?"

"Got it."

"Varsity player. Not a star, maybe not even a starter. Running back. Went into the military, either before or right after college. Not heard of since."

"My God! Pete Souza!"

"Tell me a little more."

"Great family. Portuguese. Generations of fishermen. With fisheries the way they are, they can't make it pay. Their boat usually just sits there. Pete's dad takes out an occasional whale-watching cruise or does a party run for the tourists. He works in a marine supply store. His mom still teaches math at the high school. Granddad restores and repairs old nautical and whaling gear for the museum. They've been torn up pretty bad since Pete went missing. Lots of brothers and sisters, but they're all over. The folks are empty nesters now. You found him?"

"Don't know. It would take more than three minutes to fill you in. Can I call you again and count on your help?"

"Those are dumb questions."

"That's what I hear. Give me a time and a number when you can be at a fax, receive that fax, and walk away with no one the wiser."

"I'll give you my home office number and fax. How is ten tonight? I can't tell anyone?"

"No. I may be wrong. But if it's him, he's in danger. He's pretty much lost his memory and he may have been persuaded that the people he loves are frauds, or have turned against him. To me, that sounds potentially nasty all around."

"Dr. Jordan, I've known the Souza family since I was a kid. They're good people. Dad's brother was in my class in high school. Losing Pete nearly destroyed them. They still have a yellow ribbon on … Oh, my God!"

"I believe you. Just one final question for now—did they speak Portuguese at home?"

"With his father's parents. The older folks never really assimilated. I heard Pete speaking some Portuguese with his grandpa when I sat down with his family to talk about colleges. But they didn't offer him much of a scholarship. Pete is a great kid. But he doesn't shine bright enough either in academics or sports to draw much attention. He's just an all-around great kid. He went into the service instead, to get his college money that way."

THIRTY

Joe had begged Dr. Rivers for help with the headaches, but Rivers insisted the headaches would stop once Joe's training progressed a bit further. *Maybe the bastard just didn't give a damn.*

Today's headache was his worst ever. He had no classes that afternoon. Sometimes, the headaches relented after he slept. Joe set two alarm clocks. He had to be somewhere at four.

At 3 p.m. Joe awoke with a grim sense of purpose. He slipped a slender "Texas Toothpick" folding knife into his pocket. *Enough of that fucking whore!*

He drove to a tiny lot near the building that housed the Residents' Clinic. He took an elevator to the third floor, and ducked into the men's room. He made sure the hall was empty before taking the stairs to the fifth floor. That hall was empty, too. Every door was shut. *That bitch should open her door at 3:55! Then, we'll see!*

Some weeny geek was leaving her office. "Thanks, Dr. Gilchrist. Thank you so much! I think I get it." *Thank you, Dr. Gilchrist.* Joe mocked, *Thank you? Fuck you very much!* When the elevator doors closed behind geek-boy, Joe sprinted to the recess in its door-frame and flattened himself against the elevator door. When Eve went into the ladies' room, she left her door open. Joe snuck in and lay in wait.

Eve Gilchrist returned to her office and closed the door behind her. She sat down and opened her appointment book. Suddenly, she sensed his presence. Joe leaned over her desk, his face contorted with rage. The sharp slender knife in his right hand was barely six inches from her face.

"What are you doing to me, you fuckin' bitch?"

Joe's left hand grasped her throat.

"The headaches never stop! Why are you doing this to me? Why are you torturing me day after day, year after year?"

He released her throat.

"Talk, you filthy cunt whore! Talk!" Eve started to talk, but Joe couldn't understand her words. His headache blurred his vision. He felt faint.

"Talk, or I'll mess up your face. You'll look like the dirty cunt you really are!"

Eve started to talk again—once again her words seemed garbled.

"OK, bitch!" Joe stabbed Eve's cheek, but no wound appeared. Not a drop of blood! Enraged, Joe grabbed her hair, pulled her head back to expose her throat, and stabbed at her right carotid artery. *There! There's the blood!* He stabbed again. *Where was she?*

He heard a muffled cry from the floor and raised his knife again. But his hand froze, paralyzed. Eve looked up at him, blood spurting from her neck. She reached out to him.

But her fingers wore no rings. Their nails were unpainted. The skin of her arms was dark, not Eve Gilchrist's alabaster white. How had Eve's hair gone raven black? Joe brushed aside her hair. He saw a lovely face with dark eyes that reached into the soul of his being. Her face showed no terror, only a profound sadness.

"Why, Peter? Why? We promised we'd always be together."

She collapsed. An enormous bomb went off inside Joe's head. He began to scream a scream that would never stop.

THIRTY-ONE

Marty Franks returned home to find several urgent messages from Will Rivers. Will rang again.

"Is Joe there? He didn't show."

"I don't know. I just walked in." Marty checked around. "There's stuff thrown all over the place. Some of his things are gone, but his kit is still here. It looks like he threw two alarm clocks against the wall and stomped them to pieces."

"I'll be right there."

Marty searched the apartment and nearby grounds. Nick's car was gone. He had taken some clothes, but not his kit. Every Program operative had a unique personal kit—weapons and other items useful should he be sent into action at short notice. *Well! Better he's on the run than on a rampage.*

THIRTY-TWO

"Jeff, I'm glad we can spend some time going over these tapes. I'm concerned."

"As am I."

"How would you like to proceed? These tapes are pretty impressive. The one leads directly to the other."

"Let's not start with that assumption. It's speculative and jumps—*post hoc, propter hoc.*"

"Fair enough," Ben agreed.

"We face two issues: the impact of Will's work upon the patient and your decision to take Eve off the case. We really do have to listen to the first tape together to address your concerns. But I already listened to the tape of Eve's last session. What a circus! She just couldn't get that patient under control."

What's going on here? We set up a meeting about what Will is doing, and Jeff puts Eve and me on trial?

"I agree that she couldn't get the session under control, Jeff. But how would you have contained things? What would you have done?"

Jeff thought for a few moments. Then he shrugged.

"I would have set limits and told this man that if he couldn't control himself more appropriately, he'd have to leave the office."

"Really?"

"Yeah. That's what I would have done."

"Well, between the two of us, I'm glad you didn't."

"Why not?"

"If you made Joe Morgan feel inadequate and vulnerable, he would have a field day blowing up in your face and punching you out if you kept at it."

"I don't know."

"Yeah, Jeff, you do. Safety requires taking a non-threatening stance. You're a powerful male authority figure. Play that card and you'd be in deep shit. Eve did better than you would have done under those circumstances. Criticizing her is ludicrous. Even bypassing what probably set this in motion, she gets high marks just for not making a bad situation worse."

"That's how you call it?"

"For sure. It was a no-win situation."

"OK. I was beginning to worry about her."

"You were right about her in the first place. I was wrong. She's shown real strength."

"OK. We can agree that Eve is blame-free and your course of action was completely correct. Let's move on."

"Ready for the tape?"

"Fire away."

Ben tried to convince himself there was a shred of hope. As Will's interview played, Ben noted the tape player's counter number for each interaction he considered problematic. They listened in silence, with tension building.

Finally, Jeff sighed, "Ben, I agree that Will is pouring it on pretty thick. But he's just repeating what many distinguished colleagues have said. I don't have a problem with their understanding."

Ben remained expressionless. He scanned his list of problematic interactions, rewound the tape to one, and let it play. Will spoke first:

> *And I wish you the best in that project, Joe. But it does cause me some concerns.*
>
> *Concerns?*
>
> *Why, yes. You know, Joe, memory is not a tape recorder. It's not like if we push the right button on the right place on the right tape, out comes your past.*
>
> *No?*
>
> *No. As a matter of fact, most responsible scholars are very cautious about trusting memory. Since it's not just there like a tape, when we go for memory we may get a confusing grab bag of fact, fiction, and encouraged imagination.*
>
> *So what comes up may not be true?*
>
> *Yes, indeed. That's why many of us who are true scientists worry about whether therapies designed to uncover the past, however good their intentions, may cause more harm than good.*

"He just threw her under the bus, Jeff! He just threw her under the bus! He shares a gratuitous concern about memory, and then uses terms like 'most responsible scholars' and 'true scientists' to characterize those whom he alleges are the better kind of people, people who wouldn't treat Joe Morgan that way."

Jeff shook his head. "Sorry. I don't see it that way."

Ben's jaw dropped. As they continued their review, Jeff found ingenious strategies to defend whatever Will said. Ben finally played Will's last outrageous remarks.

Well, perhaps I overstated my case, Joe. I feel very strongly about protecting patients from bad treatment. Maybe I become too much of a crusader.

"He might as well have been saying that Eve, and that I, and you for that matter, are dangerous and misguided people he wishes he could stop from doing our dastardly deeds at the expense of the vulnerable."

"That's not how I see it, Ben. He's voicing reasonable and well-respected opinions."

"Let's summarize, Jeff. Resident's supervisor sends resident to consultant. Distinguished scholar says resident treating patient is doing patient wrong and expert consultant is bogus. Resident's supervisor doubts merits of resident, questions consultant's perspective, and demonstrates profound dissociative symptoms."

"Dissociative symptoms?"

"The supervisor has apparently dissociated that he asked that very consultant to become involved so the consultant could do or teach resident to do exactly what distinguished scholar says is oh, so very, very bad!

"You may want to talk to that supervisor, Jeff. Give him a piece of your mind! Tell him that a distinguished scholar said that if he supports stuff like he recommended there must be something very, very wrong with him!"

THIRTY-THREE

Marty and Will sat in a secluded alcove at the Faculty Club, too preoccupied to put up the pretense of polite conversation. Finally, Jerry delivered their coffee, and Will turned to Marty.

"Marty, what the hell is happening?"

"I don't know. I've reviewed his whole file. Only two things stand out."

"I know," said Will. "Headaches and the girl he left behind him, the girl we've tried to convince him is dead, the girl we've been trying to convince him was a whore, the girl we've tried to blot out of his memory for years now, and the headaches. The fucking wuss can't handle the headaches!"

"I know you don't want to hear this, Will, but I just don't think we can leave the Nicks in so much pain. Their headaches really get in the way. I covered Nick W. one weekend. He spent the whole time in a darkened room with three ice bags on his head."

"Until you get your degree and demonstrate you're some hot-shit psychologist, do me the favor of shutting your fucking mouth! Those headaches will stop when the training is complete."

"But …"

"That's it! Let's move on."

Marty Franks bit his tongue. In the Program, subordinates were encouraged to voice their disagreements—once. The next moves remained the prerogative of superiors. Marty had voiced his dissent. Pushing things further would serve no purpose.

"Your heart is in the right place." Will was pushing himself to be more humane, but feigning conscience or concern strained his emotional resources.

"We want to be as kind as we can. In the long run, the Nicks are best served by mastering their programs. Some of these decisions were made far above my head, Marty. I trust our chain of command. I'd like to think I'm the sharpest fellow around, but we both know that's not so."

One of us does, you conceited prick!

"We follow Johnson's lead, and who knows who calls the shots for Johnson? The top folks will be watching us and what we do like hawks.

"Joe Morgan, our Nick Gregorides, is in the wind. He's run off after a period of increasing distress in connection with his seeking treatment outside the Program, a complete violation of protocol. I'm hinting to my chair that his treatment is inappropriate and potentially destabilizing. Bottom line? We really don't know why."

Marty Franks labored to keep his composure. *This is on you! The Program is sadistic, but we all bought in to that. But you take it a step too far. Why do you think I can't see through you? Or is it that you can't see through yourself?*

"Well, where does that leave us, Will? You know I'll follow your lead. I'm not sure how to proceed." *That should satisfy this smug fucker!*

"Let's kick things around. Then I'll boil it down and bring Johnson into the picture."

Gradually both pushed themselves beyond their mutual misgivings. They had to keep a united front.

Johnson was advised that Nick Gregorides was missing, and given a somewhat inflated picture of their efforts and the obstacles they had encountered. They suggested several possible courses of action. All involved efforts to obtain information from the records of Dr. Gilchrist and Dr. Jordan, or interrogating them directly. Will suggested eliminating Ben Jordan.

THIRTY-FOUR

Joe Morgan left US 95 at Mystic, Connecticut, filled his tank, and drove into Mystic Seaport's historic park. Something drew him to the restored old ships and harbor buildings. The noise of happy people intrigued him. He began to feel young and small. Joe fell in with a crowd of tourists being conducted through the ships by guides dressed in costumes from whaling days. He became absorbed in watching whaleboat crews drill and demonstrate their maneuvers. They reenacted how the whaleboats of another era brought the harpooner alongside a whale, and how the lines were handled once the whale was harpooned.

Joe felt smaller and younger still. A strong hand rested gently on his left shoulder. A dark and weathered forearm to his right pointed toward the boats. He heard a whisper in his right ear. It didn't seem to speak English, but he understood.

"So you see, Peter, the boat has a pointy bow and a pointy stern. They could go quick in the other direction. They'd be safe in a following sea. Now look—see what the man is holding up now? That's a harpoon …"

As long as Joe heard this strange voice, his headache just wasn't there. As the headache resumed, Joe cried inside his mind, *Whoever you are! Please come back!* Then, he heard a little boy's voice. Again, the language seemed strange, but he understood.

"Did you ever have a harpoon, Grandpa?"

"When I went to sea, Peter, they fired harpoons from a gun like a cannon. But my Papa taught me how to throw a harpoon when I was a boy. The real old captains worried, 'What if that gun breaks down when we're among the whales?' So they hired an old-fashioned harpooner or two, just in case. And yes, one day I was below decks when I heard 'Bang!!!' an' then the loudest cussin' I ever heard. Right after that, captain begins shouting, 'Silva! Silva! Boat One! Souza! Souza! Boat Two! Make ready to lower away! Make ready to …'"

Then the voice was gone and the incredible headache returned. But for a few brief moments, Joe Morgan was suffused with innocent joy and happiness—precious, unfamiliar, and gone all too soon.

* * *

Joe realized that he must have been standing in one place for quite a while. The press of one group of tourists after another watching one fascinating whaleboat and harpoon show after another disguised his statue-like immobility. He shook off a profound unwillingness to move, made his way to his car, and reluctantly started to drive.

He headed toward the water and followed the shore as he drove north, retreating to US 1 North when no roads ran closer to the sea. Reaching Stonington, he parked close to the harbor. Walking along a pier where commercial fishermen still docked, his headache left him.

A boat was unloading the day's catch. Mercedes and Cadillacs driven by well-dressed men and women pulled up to the pier. The drivers turned on their flashers and stepped out to buy fresh fish right at dockside. Orders for nearby markets and restaurants were assembled and offloaded into ice-filled chests and baskets.

Why am I so hungry? I'm a steak and potatoes guy. Joe wondered that all the way to his table in a seafood restaurant overlooking the piers, a restaurant so far above his budget that he feared he'd be eating bread and water for a month. By the time Joe finished a feast of clams, salad, and an incredible tuna steak, he was pleased with his investment.

Lingering over a second beer, Joe looked away from the pier and glanced around the restaurant. He finally noticed the other diners. *What's wrong with me? I'm acting like some bozo! An old granny could have crept up with a walker and stabbed me in the back. Oh, fuck it!*

No diners stirred his interest or his apprehension. Turning back to enjoy his view of the pier area, Joe relished the beauty of multicolored lights reflecting across the water as darkness fell. A lovely young woman walked along the quay. She waved. A young man waved back as he walked toward her.

They kissed politely. The boy looked around, saw no one looking, and embraced her more passionately. She responded briefly before giggling and pushed him away.

Joe felt soft lips on his own. He tasted salt on his tongue. Was that sand between his toes? He blinked. *Yes, I'm in this restaurant. But it's like I'm somewhere else, too.*

After leaving Stonington, he continued north. His headache began to return. He fought to push on, but he didn't know where he was going. He lost some time, recovering himself on Rhode Island 138 near the campus of the state university. He realized he must have returned to 95 and then turned off again. Pushing on, signs indicated 138 would intersect US 1. At a service station at their junction, he gassed up and asked if there was a decent cheap motel nearby.

Disciplined to get optimal exercise and sleep, Joe rarely watched late night TV. *But this Johnny Carson guy was a hoot!* An air-headed guest earned a classic Carson double take, and the audience roared. That reminded him unpleasantly of his own memory problems. He switched channels, but came right back to Carson, now dressed in a robe and turban as Carnac the Magnificent, cracking up the audience. *Too good to miss! What else has passed me by?*

* * *

Across the Nile, an endless file of laborers struggled with long heavy lines to move large limestone blocks, girdled about with protective mats, over lubricated rollers. They advanced so slowly that they barely seemed to move at all. Along the shore grew a dense growth of bulrushes, soon to be harvested and processed into sheets of papyrus for scholars and scribes. It drew the attention of a couple that strolled together, enjoying the scene.

A powerfully built male figure with a fantastic beaked head walked down to the shore. Pushing back some reeds, he pointed toward the water. A graceful young woman, slender and dark-haired, leaned over to look, one hand protecting an elegant golden diadem, ringed round with colorful gemstones. It seemed so natural, so expectable, for such gems to adorn a person so regal. Hundreds of tiny little fish, recent hatchlings, had taken shelter among the reeds. The male scooped up a few in his cupped hands, and held them up for her to see more closely. They smiled at one another. Gently and lovingly, he placed the tiny fish back among the reeds.

"Soon enough, Seth," she said, "we will have a family of our own."

And did that beaked face turn into his own? Maybe briefly. But then a man who wore a laurel wreath appeared. He stood tall in his chariot, passing beneath a triumphal arch in Rome. He saluted a lovely patrician woman, who smiled and put her hand over her heart as he passed, watching him with loving eyes as the long procession snaked its way into the Forum. For a moment, had he seen himself in that chariot?

Another scene. A Greek warrior chieftain oversaw his men pulling his dark ship onto the sandy beach of their homeland, the shore they left behind when they went to war many months before. Only when his duties were completed would he permit himself to turn toward the fields just up from the landing. A graceful dark-haired woman stood on a small rise, trying to restrain a host of screaming children from rushing toward him. He started to pull himself into the posture of the famous general that he was, to strike a pose of military bearing that would proclaim his stature and his power—for a fraction of a second. Then, throwing dignity and decorum to the four winds and the blue Aegean sky, he cried out the names of his wife and his children and rushed toward them even faster than he had charged the ranks of his enemies. Man, wife and children collapsed in one delirious, laughing, crying mass. "I'm home!" he screamed to the great ones in Olympus. "I'm home!"

Joe's own face turned to kiss a wife he knew was his ....

Joe felt sand beneath his feet. He held a slim soft hand in his own. He awakened startled, confused, and desperately trying to hold on to the joy of that Greek warrior. *Who was he? Who was she? Who were they?*

A disembodied voice floated toward him, carried by an unsensed breeze. Softly, it said:

"Nerine."

THIRTY-FIVE

The following day, Will, Ben, and Jeff met far from other offices and ears. Will's outbursts exploded like cannon shells at point blank range. Ben, relaxed to the point of insolence, seemed unaffected, provoking Will to do his worst.

Jeff made heroic but futile efforts to create a conciliatory atmosphere. Will Rivers, preeminent scientist and scholar, had become a human volcano, but his invectives rolled off Ben Jordan like water off a duck's back.

This was the nightmare scenario Bill Darymple had warned Jeff to avoid.

"You may want to leave, Ben. You won't like what I have to say. But it has to be said."

"Please go on. It will be a lovely change to be stabbed in my chest instead of my back."

"How do you put up with this sarcastic bastard?"

Will took a deep dramatic sigh. Then he turned to face Jeff.

Ben's calmness had become unnatural, almost frightening.

"You know, Ben has been beating the drum that I don't do clinical work. But just because I don't practice doesn't mean that I don't work with people. I interview maybe up to half a dozen subjects some days. Full work-ups to screen subjects.

I do follow-ups after certain protocols. If subjects are upset, I deal with them."

Jeff came in carefully. "So, Will, you have a lot of contact time with your subjects? Ben, he spends more time with folks than I do. A lot of what he does sounds like clinical work."

Ben said nothing.

"Jeff gets it, Ben. Hell, some days I spend more time with people than you do."

Will continued, "Ben, you do a lot of clinical work, and I hear it's good work by and large."

Score a few points, Will, Jeff rooted. *Force Ben to make concessions.*

Will continued: "But you have no claim to objectivity, Ben. I do, you don't."

"What do you mean?" Jeff wanted Will to make a strong showing, but Will had suddenly veered in an unexpected direction.

"I didn't want to share this. Ben, you suspected that some of our grants were government grants. You're right. And some of those Glenville-Rodgers folks, like you suspected, work with military intelligence. They know about you, Ben. About your military experience, about how you lost your wings over in Israel."

"Lost his wings?"

"Ben was a pilot. He was captured. He broke down during interrogation. They were afraid he'd turned, so they wouldn't let him back in the air. You want to deny any of that, Ben?"

Ben contained himself, but Will had scored a hit. *How could Will know about incidents Israeli military and intelligence services had suppressed?*

Interrogation? No, torture. Ben was forced to watch two of his men destroyed in front of him. Anguish drove most of that terrible week out of his memory, but shards and fragments, often too brief and disintegrated to grasp, bedeviled him day and night.

"Sure I want to. But some is true, some is false, and some … Who knows?"

"This comes from American military intelligence sources."

"Tell them to do their homework."

"I don't know what to think, Ben," said Jeff.

"I was a pilot in Israel. I did not lose my wings. I was on detached duty when I was captured during a counterterrorism operation that went bad. I never returned to flight status."

"What about breaking down?"

"Sorry. There is something about a week of torture that's kind of unfriendly to one's memory. I don't remember very much."

"So, that's what I mean, Jeff," Will pressed his attack, "When it comes to dealing with a patient who may have suffered something like what Ben suffered and can't remember, Jeff, I doubt that he can be objective." Will did his overly dramatic sigh once more, but now Jeff was listening.

"When it comes to this sort of thing, Jeff, Ben is a broken man. Why do you think I butted in in the first place? My research is relevant. It may be of help. But I knew right off that Ben would come into this with real countertransference problems, and that's not good for Eve's patient. I mean, your patient, Jeff. I knew that if you knew this stuff, you would pull Ben off the case.

"I didn't want to stab Ben in the back, no matter what he thinks. I tried to finesse the situation. I tried to take the high road with science. But, as time goes on, and I hear this paranoid stuff coming back at me, I have to speak up. Sorry, Ben. You shouldn't be anywhere near this case.

"Jeff, play it any way you see fit. But I strongly recommend that you persuade Ben to back off. He's the one who's endangering that patient's safety."

Calm and controlled at last, Will excused himself and left quietly. He had completed the mission assigned to him, and delivered the bomb crafted by Johnson's superiors.

"Another great exit. I gotta learn me some of those moves." Ben shifted in his chair, now more professional and focused.

"Let's review a few things. Remember when Will first butted in?"

"Offered his help?"

"Butted in. You said he asked about the 'guy.'"

"Yeah."

"How did he know it was a guy? You bent over backwards to be gender neutral."

"I don't know how significant that is, Ben."

"Will tried to pump Eve for information. Check that out with her. She held the line about what she understood she had to hold back, but he led her into enough for him to figure a few things out. He told her that he had to know certain things because he had to be able to account for his time and pay back his grant for 'time away.' You know that's bullshit, but most residents wouldn't."

"It is bullshit, but is that important? Don't you think he was just being anal?"

"A lot of things are anal … But why be gross about what an asshole he is?"

"Ben!"

"Jeff, Will teaches two courses and a research seminar. He has two dissertation students in the department of psychology, where he's also a professor. He draws no salary for that. His grant couldn't possibly have the stipulations he lied about. The courses and seminar are right out there in the U's bulletin, right there in public, not like some quick consultation that could be overlooked or rationalized. He lied to Eve and played her to get information, and he played you."

"That's troubling. It really is. But I have to tell you that rather than draw dire implications, I'm inclined to think Will tends toward sneaky, and you tend toward paranoid. I'm upset with both of you."

"You should be concerned. But begin by remembering what a pain in the ass I am when it comes to coverage schedules. You lose me one weekend a month, for weeks every summer, and during deployments. In all this rush of Will-full bullshit you seem to forget that I fly C-141 Starlifters for the New Jersey Air National Guard. When I do, I am Colonel Benjamin Jordan. America trusts me with planes worth tens of millions of dollars. The Air Force thinks I can be responsible for the well-being of my crew and for the lives of over 120 fighting men when we transport troops. Will should be so broken and unreliable! I know you and he are close. I know he's our shining star, and I know that some of the issues he raises could have substance. I know, and I'm sure that you know, that there is something going on that I don't know about. Maybe once you didn't know about it either. I wouldn't put it past Will to try to intimidate people. I just wish I knew why, and what the hell is going on. I accept that the world is a complicated place, too damn often a nasty hurtful place, and that most things are shades of gray … Nothing new about that. But someone, someone who couldn't have acted alone, did something completely evil to that kid.

"Here is where Will was more on target than he knew. Sure. What happened nearly destroyed me. The men who saved me were sworn enemies, but honorable warriors. They wouldn't condone what was happening. They put their lives on the line to bring what was left of me back to the IDF under a white flag. I can't do any less for Eve's patient. In some crazy way, just like me, this man has been left behind enemy lines, even if those lines are screwed up American lines. Don't think I'll do anything less."

"Shit, Ben! Can't anything be uncomplicated? I could use some simple black and white issues where I can make a clean decision and come away feeling I've done the right thing." Jeff paused.

"Ben? A question …"

"Maybe."

"Is that why your son has an Islamic middle name?"

"Classified. But I have always respected your intelligence … When you use it. It upsets me when you refuse to put it to work."

Ben started to leave the room. Then he turned back.

"Jeff, did you notice any significant omissions from Will's list of my sins and shortcomings."

"Just that you make lousy puns. Why?"

"Put yourself in Will's place and make a case that I'm some sort of bozo. Where would you start?"

"Let me think. So much to say, so little time. Well, I guess I would tell you that a resident following your plan of treatment was almost killed by a patient whose treatment you were consulting to and partially directing. I would tell you that for the well-being of everyone, including yourself, I was taking you off the case and would have some independent experts evaluate the situation and give me their feedback before I took another step."

"Right! Every reservation you're raising is solid. But good thinking like that was strangely absent from Will's rant. He came here on a mission that had nothing to do with the clinical situation. He hasn't heard the recent tapes. He's made the same theoretical arguments over and over, and now he's progressed to personal attacks. He's lied about when he learned certain things. He can't keep his facts straight.

"And you know I have information and witnesses to challenge things Will said. Now, Will says I lost my wings. You know I'm still flying. You said nothing."

Ben kept eye contact with Jeff through a prolonged silence. Finally, Jeff looked away, shrugged, and caught Ben's eyes again.

"Sometimes, Ben, I have to make the decisions that are best for the whole department, the Med School, and the whole U. This is one of those times. I'm not happy, but it's the job I'm paid to do."

"So, I guess you never knew about the camps and the box cars?"

"That's pretty damn low, Ben."

"Not from where I stand. You're too good a person to handle things this way."

THIRTY-SIX

Jeff reviewed the battle. Will was no clinician. To talk to people is one thing. To be responsible for their care is a different affair. Will had neither the heart nor the soul of a healer. But if Ben was bringing irrationality into his work, however well disguised, that could be a major problem.

Jeff couldn't shake off Ben's rebukes. He knew he deserved them, but he wanted Ben to let him off the hook. *Ben should know I had to do what I had to do.*

Jeff tried to think through what had to happen. Will would be satisfied if Ben was off the case. Ben would never be satisfied unless Will was off the case. Eve had to be kept from harm. Joe Morgan needed effective treatment. A really great chairman should be able come up with a brilliant creative solution. But his mind remained depressingly blank and barren.

He opened a locked drawer in his desk and pulled out a bottle of sixteen-year-old Highland Park Scotch. Highland Park was one of the few things Will and Ben agreed about. Each had given him a bottle at one time or another.

Jeff celebrated each and every sip of the single malt. After an inch or so, a notion began to creep into his mind. He poured a quarter inch more, and began to entertain the notion that he might be a really great chairman after all. Jeff had suddenly remembered Raymond T. Hawkes, M.D., a.k.a. the Leper.

* * *

"Ray, do you have a few minutes?"

The Leper scanned his empty appointment book.

"Of course, Jeff. What's up?" *I have a few hours, Jeff, even a few days to spare in lovely Devils' Island North.*

"I'm sure you've noticed the difficult situation that's been developing."

"No, Jeff. I haven't." *In my isolated little outpost, the department could blow itself to smithereens, and I wouldn't know it for a month or so. In fact, my office would be the safest place to be at the end of the world. You'd never know it happened! You would live forever!*

"I think you can help me solve a problem. There's a patient Will Rivers and Ben Jordan are going to war about. I want to throw this hot potato to you."

"To me?"

"It involves an ex-military guy probably exposed to some brainwashing process that used hypnosis and conditioning. Ben thinks Will is intruding where he doesn't belong. Will thinks Ben has major countertransference issues. Eve Gilchrist is the resident, stuck in the middle. I need to take those two out of the picture. All Will seems to want is to get Ben off the case, but Ben doesn't want to back off. Ben thinks highly of you. I'm hoping Ben trusts you enough to step aside if he knows things are in your hands."

"Jeff, this is complicated."

"I'm not asking. I need you to do this."

"Like a direct order?"

"That's it. Look, Ray. You know your stuff and you have high principles, sometimes high enough to do you a disservice. I can't push Will to the brink. The department can't afford to lose him. I'd hate to lose Ben. But I can afford to. If I can't put out this fire and someone gets burned, it won't be Will. Please do your friend a favor."

"You got it, chief. But I'll be away for a few days."

"This can hold that long. Thanks, Ray. By the way, we anticipate some shuffling about with graduations, retirements, and there's a rumor someone's moving on. I told Sheila to move you back over ASAP. Weisel meant well, but he missed the big picture.

"I haven't told Jordan yet. I'm still trying to work out how to do this. For now, familiarize yourself with the case, but don't discuss this or take any steps."

Ray leaned back in his chair. His head made a loud thud as it hit the wall behind him.

I just lost my house in this divorce from hell. Ben's letting me crash in his carriage house. Does Jeff think he can sweet-talk me into buddy-fucking Ben? What the hell am I supposed to do now?

THIRTY-SEVEN

Johnson met Will and Marty at the Four Seasons Hotel in downtown Philadelphia. Others held out a carrot at the end of a stick. Johnson front-loaded his operatives with carrots. Tonight's carrot was dinner at the Fountain Restaurant. He worked like a drug dealer, offering free samples to new customers until they become addicted and desperate to get more and more and more.

"We don't know where Nick is, or where he is headed. Given how we've trained him, the possibilities are endless.

"You've done a masterful job, Will! You've backed Jeff Kane into a corner. I'm glad Eve Gilchrist is off the case. Pretty women can be quite disruptive. Ben Jordan is compromised, but remains a problem.

"We have to consider who might have information we can use. If someone does, how can we extract it? General surveillance is in place at locations where intelligence thinks Nick might show. They'll do the zone defense, so to speak. We have to do the man to man. Any thoughts, Will?"

"Every contact with Nick as Joe Morgan was taped for training purposes, Mike."

"Can we acquire that information?"

Will handed Johnson a bulky manila envelope.

"Copies of his interviews with both Dr. Gilchrist and myself. Tapes and transcripts. My analysis is included."

"You sure went the extra mile. Well done."

He turned to Marty.

"However this goes down, Marty, know this doesn't reflect poorly on you. We made certain estimates about how much coverage we would need. We never anticipated having to keep these fellows on a short leash. If we have to, the project will be untenable in the long run.

"This Gilchrist girl seems to have reached past some of our conditioning, and from what Will says, this Jordan guy is loaded for bear. This is our first encounter with an outsider with sophisticated knowledge about what we do. That leaves us two problems to solve. First, we have to locate Nick Gregorides and either bring him back in or eliminate him and any problems he could pose. Second, we have to learn what Gilchrist and Jordan know, and get them out of the picture. Jordan may be someone we'll need to deal with sooner or later.

"Will, step to the sidelines. We can't risk them making you. First we're going to have to get Gilchrist's notes, if any, and ask her a few questions. Marty, you'll team with another operative we'll bring in. We'll have to go after Gilchrist first, and soon."

"What about Jordan?"

"We can't be definitive about him until we interrogate Gilchrist. Where can we reach her?"

"She lives in a townhouse in Bryn Mawr," Marty offered. "Her entryway is pretty secluded. Kill a few of the outer lights and we have a good shot."

"No! We'll send a locksmith and security systems guy we use to check the place out and make us some keys during the day. He'll bypass parts of the alarm system. It will look like it works, but nothing will happen if she hits the panic button or other emergency signals. He can do some work on Jordan's place, too."

He looked to Marty.

"You'll back up a man who'll bring something new in the way of persuasion, capsaicin."

Will decided he couldn't fake it. "I don't get it," he admitted.

"Short version, Will," Johnson explained. "That's the active ingredient that makes hot peppers hot and pepper spray effective. Some of the sadists and the bad-ass militias south of the border get a kick out of dousing a woman's vagina, anus, whatever, with really potent stuff. It's agony. We have the most powerful preparation around. If you use it, you're going to make one hell of an impression on that very special lady."

They all chuckled. Will instantly saw an image of Eve Gilchrist tied down, spreadeagled, completely naked, writhing, her pelvis churning as she struggled to escape the ruthless pain. He imagined her screaming, begging him for the relief he would never grant. He hoped his colleagues didn't notice his erection. *Too bad I won't be there to see it!*

THIRTY-EIGHT

"Eve, you're young. You have youth's irrational belief that you're invulnerable and immortal, reality be damned. You are not safe!"

"Don't you think you're a tad paternalistic, Ben?"

"No! When it comes to you and the other residents, I'm over the top paternalistic. Things are going crazy, and I can't seem to convince you or anybody else to take me seriously."

"What about you, Dr. Jordan? If there are bad guys, I'm not the brain trust they have to worry about. Now, if this is really about dressing well, and they're after my fashion secrets, I've got you by a country mile."

Ben wasn't chuckling.

"Bad joke?"

"These people seem to think you're the easier target. Joe's been set up to drive you away. Pragmatically, that actually may be calculated to make everyone else back away from Joe Morgan to protect you. And that's what has to happen. Ideally, I should take over Joe's treatment, but the way Will seems to be pulling Jeff's strings, I doubt that can happen."

"I didn't want to be protected. Joe is my case!"

"Was your case. Where are your parents now?"

"I don't want them involved."

"Understood, but from where I sit, a few weeks overseas behind embassy walls guarded by Marines looks safer than walking across campus. I have friends overseas. I could probably get you a good elective in a cool place. Jeff would back that."

"I spent my childhood under guard! No way! Look, Dr. Jordan. My folks are on vacation, cruising up to the Vineyard. You think I'd be safe with two old alcoholics on a sailboat? Get real! Sure, my parents are into hunting and shooting. If I were being stalked by a nasty deer or menaced by a malevolent flock of clay pigeons, they'd be my salvation. Beyond that? Hah!"

"OK. I have a few ideas."

"Forget about it."

Lisa Hart stuck her head into the office.

"Hey, Lisa."

"Hi, Dr. Hart."

"This isn't the time, I see. But Ben, I wanted you to know … six weeks in, and all's well. Details later."

"I'm glad the unknown resident is doing better," said Eve.

"Whoa!" Ben cried.

Lisa laughed, "Ben, Eve is pretty smart. Am I correct that you pulled that out of your, uh, feminine intuition, and that there was no breach of confidentiality?"

"Nope! Let's remove the gender bias, Lisa. Simple logic. It stands to reason that Ben would want to hover over the individual who got into a bad place, but he'd figure that having the big dog himself sniffing around would be too intimidating. Ergo, Ben would arrange a proxy watchdog, probably someone likely to think and feel the way he does. My guess? Dr. Liebowitz or Dr. Hart. Sorry, Lisa!"

Lisa Hart's laughter had a wonderful silvery quality.

"Proxy watchdog! I've been called worse!"

"Glad you dropped by, Lisa! Let me give you a hypothetical."

"OK."

"Imagine this: A man seeks therapy from well-regarded Pooh-Bah Lisa Hart. Through no fault of Dr. Hart's, the patient's reality-testing crumbles. Sometimes he perceives her as someone else with whom he has an intense love-hate relationship. He loves and desires her, but rages against her because he's sure she betrayed him. In session he attacks Dr. Hart with irrational accusations and unfair criticisms. Finally, he grabs his chart, throws it against the wall, trashes her office, and slams her door so hard that one of its hinges tears out.

"Does Dr. Hart lope along, business as usual? Or does she conclude that proceeding with the case is unwise, behave with caution, and maybe even permit herself to be protected for a while?"

"And how old is the wise and wonderful Dr. Hart in this scenario?"

"What does that have to do with it?" Eve asked.

"Everything! If I were still young and green, Eve, I wouldn't take it seriously. If I were a little less young, but still young, mind you, I would remind myself that for being attacked on the job, mental health workers rank just behind convenience store clerks and taxi drivers. I might try to convince myself I was safe, and just humoring someone else, like my husband, but I wouldn't continue. And if I thought I might be stalked, I'd stay somewhere else for a while, try to carpool in and out, and never walk alone."

"He didn't pay you? He didn't have you lying in wait outside?" Eve teased.

"Let's cut to the chase, Eve." Lisa turned dead serious. "You're entering one of the lowest-paying and least respected medical specialties. Psychiatrists start out a bit masochistic.

"Given our field's baseline acceptance of self-sacrifice and toleration of pain and stress, and late adolescents' and young adults' sense of grandiose invulnerability, I'd say the very young Professor Hart would defy Ben's common sense and argue him into the ground. She would call him paternalistic and authoritarian.

"But, a very few years later, she'd accept his advice, bitching, moaning, and groaning every step of the way."

"Traitor!" said Eve.

"Pack some stuff. You can stay with my tribe for a few days."

She checked her watch.

"Speaking of kids, I'm out of here. This card has my home info. I have to pick up the kids from day care. Dinner is whenever I finish making it, I'll guess seven. You have a lot of time to get to toddler land. Pack old stuff or things that don't stain. I'm gone."

God! That woman is class! Ben mouthed "Thank you!" as Lisa made her exit.

"I'll pay her back! I'll pack a steamer trunk."

THIRTY-NINE

The white van's logo read, *James O'Brien & Sons—Main Line Locksmiths.* Its handsome young driver wore a dark green uniform. His bright green shamrock-shaped nametag identified him as James O'Brien, Jr.

"Junior" O'Brien found Louie, the maintenance man at Eve's complex.

"You're not the usual guy."

"Right you are, Louie. This ain' our usual territory. We're out of Devon, further out. And I hope your usual guy won't be pissed. But, you know, I'm sure he'd understand. You see, Miss Gilchrist—it's so hard to call someone you knew since she was a kid Doctor Gilchrist—ah, her dad's cousin is married to my dad's brother. So, when she told her dad—they talk every day, you know—when she told her dad she must have dropped her keys goin' from her car to her office, he called his cousin to get our number, you know, figuring family would be quicker. Few more calls and Dad says, 'Junior'—I hate that—thirty-three and still 'Junior'—he says, 'Junior, hop over there and fix up Miss Gilchrist's problem.'"

"Waste of your time and effort. I've got a spare I can leave for her."

"Tell you what, Louie. Let me copy your spare. I'll make a few dups and leave 'em with you."

"Well, I quit at four. I gotta keep an eye on things."

"Right you are. Thirty minutes, I promise. I'll run one down to her, return yours plus a couple, and leave what she wanted on her kitchen counter."

"Still a waste of your time ..."

"Hey. The old man has a hard head. He knows only one answer—'yes.'"

"Mine, too. Yeah. OK. I'll be right back."

* * *

Half an hour later, Junior handed Louie an envelope with his original and two copies. When Louie checked, an envelope with four bright new keys, marked "Dr. Gilchrist," sat on Eve's counter.

Junior delivered several copies of Eve's key to Johnson.

"She gotta be rich. Lots of people have reproductions of what she's got, but all of hers are artists' prints—signed and numbered! A Monet, a Picasso, and a Mondrian. I fixed her security system. And whatever goes in or out of Jordan's house, it's covered."

FORTY

Junior returned to Eve's place driving a Mercedes. Now he wore designer jeans, a silk shirt, a light leather jacket, and sunglasses. A red Phillies cap, pulled low, shielded his face. He watched for any development that might complicate the Program's plans.

There she is! 4:30! Home real early! By five, Eve Gilchrist had made three trips to her car with suitcases, and two more with hanging clothes.

No way I could afford this broad!

Junior radioed in.

"We have an empty nest tonight. God knows where the kids are."

Lou answered, "Oh, well, if it's just us, let's go out." Will believed his "fiancée" had been selected to satisfy his needs and be a social asset. Actually, Lou ranked above Will, held a prestigious Australian doctorate, and was primed to replace him if he faltered.

Lou, Franks, and a man named Stein ransacked Eve's apartment looking for anything that might relate to her work with Nick or provide information that might be used to influence her. Eve Gilchrist had champagne tastes, and indulged them.

"I would kill for her wardrobe!" said Lou admiringly.

"This search is a bust." Franks was disgusted. "She seems to be a good little girl who keeps to herself. Everything on her desk schedule is professional. Months back I see weird entries about '007.' One day she wrote, 'James Bond is dead!'"

Lou guessed, "I bet that the 007 entries are Fridays and weekends."

"Yeah. They are!"

"Probably her code for a boyfriend who was into that stuff and bored her silly, so she dropped him. Move on."

There was nothing more to be found.

"OK," said Lou. "Toss her clothes. Take some underwear into the bathroom. Make it look like some pervert did something filthy with her panties. That just might make her think Joe Morgan is some sicko sex freak, and scare her off. But we still have to interrogate her."

* * *

After Eve unpacked, flabbergasting both Lisa and her husband, she realized she'd left her running gear behind. Bud Hart escorted Eve back to her place.

"Oh my God! Every bit of my clothing! Everything's been thrown around."

"I'm calling the cops."

"No! Please don't!"

Bud was as unflinchingly direct as Lisa.

"You do it, or I do it."

* * *

After Eve called the police, Bud explained things to Lisa. He chatted briefly with both children, and sang them bedtime songs. As soon as Bud hung up, Lisa tracked down Ben Jordan.

* * *

Ben spoke to the duty sergeant at the U's security office. He gave him his own name and those of Jeff, Will, and Eve, and requested their offices be checked.

The sergeant called Ben back near eleven.

"Say, Doc! As far as we can see, only one office was disturbed."

"Dr. Gilchrist's?"

"Yeah. Hey, Doc! What do you know about this?"

"I know that the four I named are involved with a case that's blowing up in our faces. Someone Dr. Gilchrist was treating. Lower Merion Police are still on site at her apartment in Bryn Mawr. Somebody trashed the place late afternoon-early evening."

"Well, her office is destroyed. Every stick of furniture is busted up, every posters is torn to shi—shreds. Somebody spray-painted a message on the wall, through a stencil. It reads 'DIE BITCH!' in capitals. We called in Philly. They're treating it as a crime scene."

Ben left Jeff a comprehensive message. He told the Harts he doubted their safety if Eve stayed a second night. The Harts agreed, sadly. They couldn't chance putting their children in harm's way. Then, Ben spoke to Eve.

"Your office at the U was trashed. Detective Bleier, Philly PD, wants to talk to you. Let the Harts take you downtown tomorrow. Let the cops take you back to the U. Park yourself in my office until I can figure out what will be safest for you."

"What about what I think?"

"And your experience arranging protection is ..."

"OK. We don't have to go there."

* * *

Ben placed a final call.

"Old Country Ornamental Plastering and Plaster Restoration. We're out of the office until tomorrow morning at nine.

Please leave a message or call back tomorrow. We look forward to serving your decorating needs."

"Ben. ASAP."

Ben's phone rang in under two minutes. He explained the situation. He was asked if Eve Gilchrist was "a nice girl, a good girl."

"Yes, Mama. She is very polite and refined." He did not say, *To a fault!* He was dealing with Mama Brazzo, and Mama Brazzo did not appreciate irony.

FORTY-ONE

When Jeff arrived, the U's new chief of security was waiting for him.

"Where were you last night, Dr. Kane?"

"I was out at a new steak place with Dr. Rivers, Dr. Brewer, my wife, and some others. Didn't make it home till after eleven, and we went to bed as soon as we got home."

"Dr. Gilchrist's office got torn apart last night. Someone sprayed, 'DIE BITCH' on her wall. Lower Merion cops were called earlier yesterday 'cause someone tossed her apartment. Is there something you want to tell me?"

"No. Nothing."

The chief was not a patient man.

"Look, Dr. Kane. I'm no psychiatrist, psychologist, whatever … But I spent over twenty years in the Navy, mostly Shore Patrol. You're holding out on me. Talk to me, or Philadelphia's finest can take you downtown and you can get squirrely with them."

"I'm the chair …"

"The president of the U ordered me to wrap this up yesterday. President trumps chair. I'm waiting."

"OK. This is clumsy."

"Should I say, 'Just the facts, ma'am,' or are you gonna run around in circles till you're downtown? Or what?"

"Two professors are battling over how to proceed with a patient Dr. Gilchrist is treating. Things have gotten out of control and we're worried about Dr. Gilchrist's safety. Dr. Jordan advised her to stay somewhere else for a while, but she didn't want any part of that."

"And this patient?"

Jeff weighed the obligations of confidentiality against the obligations to protect others from danger.

"Someone's life may be at risk, so I'll worry about confidentiality tomorrow. His name is Joe Morgan. He's ex-military. He has some weird condition and he seems to mistake the past for the present and one person for another at times."

"His diagnosis is 'some weird condition'?"

"I wish I could do better. Jordan thinks he's been brainwashed."

The chief's eyebrows raised. "I had to deal with some of those poor bastards. OK. Expect a visit from Philly. Detective Bleier caught this one. Answer his questions straight and he'll be gone in five minutes."

FORTY-TWO

Eve Gilchrist never had and never would have ventured into South Philadelphia of her own free will. Its narrow streets of row houses, Italian restaurants, markets, delis, and cheesesteak meccas were strange and unfamiliar. Stopped at a light on her way to the home of someone named Lucco Brazzo, she wanted to blow through the red light and burn rubber back to Bryn Mawr. The Coliseum, she knew. The Spanish Steps, she knew. Via Veneto, she knew. But the Mummer's Museum? The Victor Café with wait staff singing opera to the patrons? Sarcone's where Ben made weekly pilgrimages for bread and stuffed pepper poppers?

Once Ben took the residents in her year to a place deep in South Philadelphia, the Osteria Siciliano. A tall, thick man who seemed to know Ben came out to greet them. He assured the residents that their cars would be safe, and patted an unnatural bulge under his left arm. *Now, that was strange and foreign!*

Ben was concerned about her safety. He suggested that she visit a friend whose family might keep her from harm. *Safe? And what does family mean in South Philly? Why did he tell me to bring extra underwear?* Eve wondered, but realized that she really didn't want to know.

Parking was a nightmare. Finally, a dark Chevrolet Blazer pulled out of a space near the Brazzos' address, and Eve parked. She stepped out of her Volvo and began arranging herself. Eve heard a motor gunning, then the squeal of brakes. The Blazer had reversed and closed in to trap her between its passenger side and the driver's side of Eve's own car. A man in a ski mask rushed toward her. Without thinking, Eve bashed him with the heavy pocketbook she held in her left hand and threw her right fist into her attacker's face with every ounce of her strength. He faltered. She swung the bag again, hammering the top of his head. He crashed to the ground, tried to get up, staggered, and fell on his face.

A row house door swung open. A heavyset man rushed out with an extremely large revolver in his hand. The big man from that restaurant! Someone in the Blazer screamed, "Abort! Abort!" Eve's attacker struggled to his feet and lurched after the departing Blazer. It stopped and reversed. Two men jumped out and dragged him into the back seat.

Now Eve felt panic and pain. Her right palm was bleeding. Two nails had broken and gashed her hand when she landed her blow. The heavy man was already at her side, asking if she was all right. At the door of the row house stood what seemed to be the very same man, just a generation older, his hands folded behind his back. He watched the retreating Blazer until it disappeared around a corner two short blocks away. An attractive gray-haired woman was at his side. She seemed disquietingly comfortable brandishing a very large butcher's knife.

"Let's get you inside. I'm Lucco. That's my Momma and my Dad."

Introductions completed, Lucco washed and dressed Eve's injuries with professional skill.

"Medic. Rangers. 'Nam."

Before she could stop herself, Eve blurted, "Hemingway."

"Ah, yes—telegraphic style. But Hemingway also said all first drafts are shit. So, I'll start again. I was a medic in Vietnam. And this is the smallest wound I've ever treated.

"That was a nice shot, Eve! Can I call you Eve? A nice shot. But you gotta do something about the way you ..."

Eve leapt to her feet, indignant. Hands on her hips, she faced Lucco down and stormed, "What do you mean? He's on the ground! I'm standing. My form was perfect!"

"Everyone can see that, dear," said Mama Brazzo. "He's talking about the way you make your fist. He just doesn't want you to hurt your wrist if the next jaw you break is any harder than with that last *faccia di merda*."

Eve turned bright red. The laughter began. She covered her face for a moment before she collapsed on a chair, and joined the Brazzos in their hysteria.

* * *

When things were calmer, Mama Brazzo took Eve aside.

"Did you bring the extra underwear? Good. You don't understand? I'll explain." Mama rarely gave anyone a chance to respond before she continued on. Eve would get no special treatment, and no explanation.

Lucco caught Ben between appointments.

"They were laying for her right there on the street. She's really something. I think she broke some muscle's jaw with one punch and nearly knocked him out with her bag."

"Shit! This won't work. You know this kind of trouble will be bad for all of you. Everything should be safe for tonight. Tomorrow, she's out."

"We can handle it ..."

"There's something about a beautiful woman that makes even smart men like you want to promise more that they should. If you promise, you deliver. I know that. But the cost/benefit ratio here looks really bad."

"Agreed. That's what Mama and Papa think, too. Ben, what about Chicago?"

"Problem is that the bad guys may be feds or fed-connected. I won't bring trouble to my uncle."

* * *

When Mama retreated to the kitchen, Eve followed.

"Can I help?"

"Can you cook?"

Eve stood silent.

Mama looked her up and down.

"Change into real clothes, grab an apron, and we'll make dinner."

Time passed easily. Mama had interesting opinions about everything, and she was a great teacher. Eve had quick fast hands and a great palate. She followed everything Mama was doing and grasped what Mama was aiming for when Mama stopped to taste how the dishes were progressing. They enjoyed being together.

When Mama took a break and had a long chat in Italian with her sister, Eve and Lucco fell into conversation. Their strong chemistry kept declaring itself in Freudian slips. Eve abandoned her usual politesse.

"Lucco, if I was the kind of girl who played around, I could get very interested in you. But I'm incredibly old fashioned, and I don't play around."

She smiled, "Don't think for a moment that I don't recognize the real deal when it comes to men. Don't think I don't feel the real deal when it comes to men. But I am who I am. Whatever that says about me, that's me."

"Eve!" Mama Brazzo was off the phone.

Lucco took Eve's hand gently, and pressed it to his lips.

"You have a friend."

Eve hugged him quickly, and started to walk away. She turned.

"That goes both ways, Lucco."

FORTY-THREE

Most of Eve's childhood had been spent surrounded by those charged with protecting her. Yes, Ben wanted to arrange for her safety, but wasn't she finally able to make her own decisions? In the privacy of her own mind, Eve struggled, bargained, and compromised. Reasoning no one would trash her place and dare to return so soon, she left word for Ben. "I have to check on my apartment and pick up a few things. Then I'll follow your plans to the letter."

Eve drove home, waved to Louie, and went to her apartment. Moments later, Junior hailed Louie from his van. When Louie came over to chat, Marty Franks stole up behind him. Louie was quickly bound, gagged, and hidden in a dumpster.

Junior would stand guard. Marty and the interrogator would go after Eve. This man, "Johnson" for the mission, specialized in torture.

Both donned ski masks, cautiously climbed the stairs, and entered Eve's apartment using one of Junior's shiny new keys. Eve reacted quickly, but Junior had disabled her panic button. She fought like a tiger, but the men soon had her bound and gagged. "Johnson" began running water into her bathtub. While it filled, the two searched Eve's place and put her purse and briefcase near the door. When the tub was filled, Johnson produced a small box containing vials of a turbid liquid. Eve shuddered.

"Dr. Gilchrist. I will ask you a number of questions about Joe Morgan. You will answer immediately and accurately, or you will be encouraged to do so. Let me indicate the nature of the encouragement."

He took firm hold of Eve's hair and dragged her to the bathtub. He forced her to her knees and plunged her head into the water. He kept her face submerged for a full minute.

As she coughed up water and gasped for breath, he said,

"Where is Joe Morgan?"

"I don't know." Eve's family sailed. She remembered drownproofing. She took a big breath before she was forced under once again. She would spit in their faces no matter what.

"Where is Joe Morgan?"

"I don't know." Eve knew she couldn't hold her breath quite long enough, but she could make them sweat.

Eve neither could nor would say more. Her interrogators grew exasperated.

"We'll have to take her with us. Unless …"

He took one of the small vials out of the box. He put on thick rubber gloves before opening it.

"Dr. Gilchrist, this is concentrated extract from Sumerian Devil peppers. They have the highest Scoville rating in the world, three thousand units above its nearest rival. Such an extract can be applied to the most private places a woman might imagine. If the woman's hands are not restrained, she will tear herself to pieces trying to rid herself of the agony. In your case, your hands are restrained. We simply will move from one very private place to another. Please consider your options."

"I can't tell you what I don't know! Please …"

Johnson instructed Marty to hold Eve still. He put down the vial for a moment to push up her skirt and take down her underwear. They lingered over Eve's body.

"Gotta do what we gotta do," said Marty.

"A true pity ..."

A hand materialized from behind Johnson, wrenching back his head and neck. As his mouth gaped open in surprise, a second hand seized the vial and shoved it into his mouth, open end first. The intruder shoved the agonized man into Franks and kicked over him, smashing Franks's face. Before Franks struggled to his feet, the intruder turned and landed a vicious elbow strike on Johnson's head, shoved a second vial down his pants, and stomped on it, hard. Johnson howled as the Sumerian Devil extract reached his open wounds.

"You and me then, Jordan!" Marty screamed.

Ben Jordan kicked Johnson again.

"Let's see what you've got, Jordan!"

Ben said nothing. He barely moved. Franks approached cautiously before launching a combination of whirling kicks.

Ben Jordan retreated a step, moving closer to a chair and awaiting Franks's next attack. The moment Franks leaped, Ben shoved the chair toward where Franks would land. Franks came down off balance, tripped, and stumbled into Ben's heel kick to his face. A terrible crunch, cracking sounds—a tooth fell from Marty's bloodied mouth. His hands went to his face. Ben launched a combination of kicks at Marty's groin and knee, but neither caught him hard enough to do damage. Johnson staggered up and moved to attack Ben from behind.

"Get the girl," Marty screamed. Ben moved to protect Eve. Marty moved to the side, pushing a couch between them. Both charged as if they were going for Eve. When Ben fell back to protect her, they turned and ran out the door with the purse and briefcase. Ben jumped up to chase them, but Junior stood at the door, his handgun pointed in Ben's direction. Ben dove for the floor and rolled toward Eve. The three men stumbled down the stairs. Ben threw an afghan over Eve, and tried to catch his breath.

Three curious neighbors poked their heads through the open door. Ben slammed it shut in their nosy faces. He removed Eve's gag and cut the ropes that bound her. She rushed to another room, and he called 911.

Police sirens were drawing near when someone shouted. "My god! Louie's tied up in the dumpster!"

"Poor Louie," said Eve, now in slacks and a top. "He's our maintenance man."

"And those other guys?"

"All they asked was 'Where is Joe?'"

"What's most important is that you're all right. What do you have that's creamy or fatty? Some of that stuff got on me. It's really brutal."

Eve found a jar of peanut butter. Ben rubbed it all over his hands.

"Water just moves it around. You need this other kind of stuff to absorb it or neutralize it."

He worked more peanut butter onto his hands.

"Did they take anything?"

"My pocketbook and my briefcase!"

"Anything in it?"

"A letter to my folks, the books I was reading, and your crystal ball gazing."

"My predictions? Oh, shit!!!"

"Why 'Oh, shit!!!'"

"Because I think I was right. Now they know where Joe's likely to go. I'll have to get there first."

"Why were you here? I mean, thanks! But how on earth …"

"Got your message. You gotta stop scaring me."

"Is that your way of screaming at me?"

FORTY-FOUR

Marty Franks's superiors were determined to learn whatever Eve Gilchrist and Ben Jordan knew, and to recover Joe. Further interrogation would have to determine whether the surprisingly tough Eve Gilchrist had more to say.

Jordan had kicked Marty's ass. Marty would face Johnson with no more than a banged up face, a missing tooth, and a seriously mutilated ego. Worse, he would face him alone. Johnson was undergoing treatment, but Marty's dental repairs could wait. Marty promised Jordan a slow death.

* * *

Marty drove to a motel near the enormous shopping malls in King of Prussia. He entered the designated room with trepidation and placed Eve's briefcase and bag on a table. As ordered, he had left them unopened.

"Johnson is receiving medical care. As per my call, Gilchrist's interrogation was interrupted. She fought like hell and was not breaking. She may be telling the truth. Jordan stormed in. He was exceptionally fast and effective. I'm amazed Johnson got back into the fight. We went for the girl, Jordan went to protect her. Then Junior backed him off."

Mike Johnson kept his wrath to himself. He would stick to positive reinforcement if he could, but so far there was nothing positive to say. Nodding, he scrutinized Eve's possessions.

"Well, what have we here? Top of the line Coach bag. Usual lady stuff, the most expensive available, worth it or not. Beautiful briefcase, no label. Probably high-end Italian custom job from this incredible leather. Toiletries, book by Luborsky, a torrid romance, *Marie Claire, Foreign Affairs*, Hartland on hypnosis, a half-written letter to her folks. Hmm. Here's a curious envelope … 'Do Not Open Until You Are Sure!!!!'"

He shook his head. "Well, I'm sure! Let's see what's here."

Johnson opened the envelope carefully. He spread two typed pages flat on the table and began to read. Then he picked them up, sat down in a chair, and reread them slowly. He shook his head, smiled, and reread the pages again, more slowly still. Finally he looked up, amazed and elated.

"Jackpot! Ben Jordan wrote this after hearing Gilchrist's first two sessions with Nick G. This is the man, Will, you tell me is an idiot. Listen to this:

> *Your patient, utilizing available information and assuming its accuracy, skipped college and went directly into the service. Given that he is highly intelligent, but no academic all-star, we may assume that either he had the choice of enlistment or jail, was drafted, has a blue collar background and was never pointed toward college, comes from a family in which sons tend to follow their fathers into an occupation (such as farming or fishing), or was unable to obtain sufficient support or scholarships to go directly to college and hoped to do so as a benefit of serving his country. The many variations of dissociative memory phenomena, in addition to profound depersonalization, suggest a chronic complex dissociative disorder with lesions of identity and memory. Those conditions are multiple personality, atypical dissociative disorder (a grab bag), or, intriguingly but unlikely, the breakdown of the secondary identity in a fugue*

state. I do not think cyclical psychotic disorders or complex partial seizures cover the waterfront. There are hints, from his intrusive phenomena, that he left behind a girlfriend with a dark complexion who remains precious to him. The girlfriend with a dark complexion and the sugar on his toast, suggestive of Portuguese sweetbread, indicate Joe Morgan may be of Portuguese ancestry. Epidemiologically speaking, plus considering his hallucinations of sand and salt air, and his mention of sand dunes, I think Joe Morgan comes from a Portuguese family that made its living from the sea, probably by fishing, and that still retains many of the ethnic customs and cooking traditions of Portugal or the Azores. Perhaps Portuguese is still spoken at home. They live near the sea. Sandy shores are typical of Cape Cod and the Islands. Same for other areas, but they got built over. Three good places to look for such a person if the Massachusetts connections are real would be near and including Fall River-New Bedford, Cape Cod, and the islands of Martha's Vineyard and Nantucket. If the Massachusetts thing is a red herring, start working down the coast of Connecticut in towns historically associated with Portuguese immigration and Portuguese involvement in the maritime trades. Stonington still has a small commercial fishing fleet. P.S.—He mentioned an Easton Street. I once stayed at The White Elephant on Easton Street in Nantucket. There's a lighthouse nearby. When he approached the U library he saw vague hints of a taller building in addition to the Easton Street sign. That fits. Lots of sand dunes on Nantucket. It once had a vigorous fishing industry. That's what I think, weird dissociative disorder, and that's where I'd look. Nantucket.

BJ."

"Fuckin' Jordan" Will muttered.

"A valuable asset if he could be turned," Johnson mused. "Any chance?"

"No fucking way!"

"Then we'll need to take him out of the picture."

"I'll do it myself."

"Will, your hatred makes you stupid! You are very, very valuable to us, but you've underestimated Jordan at every step. Marty could trash you in a second, Will, and Jordan kicked Marty's ass. Jordan could kill you without breaking a sweat."

"But ..."

"Don't even think about it. We both read his classified file. But you read it to find things to discredit him, and I read it to understand what danger he poses. Keep your priorities straight and shove your fucking ego where the sun don't shine. We had twenty-plus men out looking for Peter Souza and they came up empty. This Ben Jordan sits on his butt and thinks for a little while ... Hear that word? Thinks!

"Marty, what you brought us probably delivers Souza on a plate. So, Will, if your ego can face it, make nice. When we take Jordan out, I don't want you to be the prime suspect."

"OK, OK. Just get him out of my face."

"If he can't be turned, he has to go. Count on it."

"Gilchrist?"

"Her family is very influential. I'm hoping that when Jordan goes down, she'll be nothing but a pretty girl with a few bruises and a wild story no one will believe. But we may have to deal with her, too."

FORTY-FIVE

Ben drove Eve and enough apparel to provide haute couture to an army of cross-dressers to Gladwyne. Elani was in Israel. His children were spending the summer with their English cousins. He would protect Eve in his own home.

Most of Lucco's childhood friends had grown up to be cops, crooks, or priests. Lucco managed his life with enough discretion to preserve his friendships with old friends on the force. Ben and Eve found two attractive but clearly formidable off-duty policewomen awaiting them in his driveway.

Lucco had briefed Officers O'Leary and Demchak. Ben did the same.

"I have no idea what's going on here. My gut and my training tell me that the best place to get the answers I need is in Massachusetts. Meantime, I need to make sure that this young lady is protected. The Lower Merion and Gladwyne police know I'm bringing you in. Let them know who's here every shift."

To Eve, Ben said,

"Back at your apartment, as soon as I realized you'd made a stupid decision, I came running. These folks will go to the wall for you. Don't put them in a bad spot with any monkey business. The bad guys are smart and dangerous. The

Gladwyne PD is small. They can't give you more than frequent drive-byes. I had to bring help on board, so here we are.

"You told me your family is into shooting, especially skeet, and you're pretty good with a light shotgun. The only shotgun here is a 12-gauge Purdey side-by-side my wife uses. Its balance is perfect. You should be quite comfortable with it."

Eve began to breathe rapidly, "But Purdeys are usually built to order. Your wife is taller than me, and I've read she's very strong."

Eve's anxiety was skyrocketing. Purdey weapons are top of the line. Most are custom built for affluent and discriminating shooters and hunters. Ben was handing Eve a weapon worth more than many of Philadelphia's old Main Line houses, and Eve knew it. She was more than a bit overwhelmed.

Ben recognized that Eve's stated misgivings were groundless. Fitting a shooter for a shotgun is mostly a matter of arm length, shoulder to wrist. Eve was a few inches shorter than Elani, but that didn't translate into major differences in arm length. Given the minimal difference in arm length involved and a weapon so well balanced that it felt almost weightless, Elani's greater height and strength were irrelevant. But Eve was apprehensive. Ben saw that rational persuasion might take more time than it was worth.

"You're right, Eve. Perhaps not the right gun for you. Neither is anything else around here. But I'll take you out back with a few shells so you'll know what to expect if you need to use it. Same with this Glock 17. It's what's here. Someone who really knows weapons is bringing something like the shotguns you've used. It should be here tomorrow."

Ben's property was large and wooded. He took Eve went to his expansive back yard. In front of a large dirt hillock, he set up cans at various ranges. Eve was adept. Even though she had never handled these weapons before, Eve nailed every can and came back on target smoothly and easily.

"I hate to leave you with strangers. Ray is crashing in the coach house down the driveway for a while. He's not due back till tomorrow. I've left him a message about all this. I can't reach him directly."

"Why can't I come too?"

"Because I think they want you off the case and me off the planet. Coming with me is a desperate move, only if we can't keep you safe here and I can't get you to stay with your parents and a million marines."

"But what has to happen for things to go back to normal? I don't want to live like this."

"Well, me neither. We need a solution that gives Nick his life back and brings the aggressive aspects of his mental illness to an end. Hopefully, a cure. Failing that, hospitalization or death. He can't be allowed to hurt you."

"Ouch!"

"Whatever is going on with Will, he needs a punch in the nose he'll never forget. And anyone else involved in this nightmare—cure 'em, contain 'em, kill 'em, or drive them off so they stay at a safe distance."

After Ben left, Eve studied both weapons. She loaded and unloaded them with eyes open, and blindfolded. She practiced grabbing either gun and bringing it to bear on a target, even whirling toward targets behind her. She finished by getting the feel of bringing the Purdey to bear at hip level. Finally, she thought through how she would approach Ben's home if she were the one planning an intrusion.

You taught me well, Uncle Buck! She recalled a glorious day in the desert with "Uncle Buck," the Marine embassy guard who accompanied her when her father served in crisis-torn lands and she needed protection. One night, before her father slid completely into his customary quiet drunken state, he told Buck he thought it would be a good thing for nine-year-old Eve to learn how to shoot. "So, take care of it," he ordered. Buck did.

Little "Cricket," as she was called, slaughtered dozens of tin cans on that bright and cloudless day. That evening Buck informed Eve's father—"The Cricket is a 'natural.'"

But that was the evening after the morning after the night before. Ambassador Gilchrist had forgotten giving this order to Buck, and ranted until others who had heard her father's order and had less to drink found the courage to come to his rescue. Ambassador Gilchrist swallowed his pride and apologized then and there. Eve enjoyed her shooting lessons until circumstances deteriorated and embassy dependents had to be evacuated. The last time she saw Uncle Buck ... Had it been that long? So many years ago! *Oh, Uncle Buck! I wish you were here!*

Eve contemplated the Purdey, a masterpiece of functionality and aesthetics. The quality of the engraving astonished her. Eve remembered this model from her family's visit to Purdey's London Gunroom on South Audley Street. Her father was there to inspect the .470 Nitro Express and other "dangerous game guns." Meanwhile, Eve and her mother admired the shotguns while the other children took a walk. Her mother was impressed, "It's just too beautiful to take into the bush. I'd be afraid to nick it or scratch it up. It's like some amazing cake so lovely that you hate to cut it up and eat it! Purdeys are works of art."

And I may have to defend myself with a masterpiece!

FORTY-SIX

"Hi, Mama! It's Ben. "Is Lucco there?"

"No, Benny. I sent him over to Sarcone's for some pepper poppers. His father makes them disappear before I can turn around. Lucco told me about the young lady."

Only Mama Brazzo called Ben "Benny." He was wise enough to leave that unchallenged.

"I need a favor. Would you mind flying that underwear she left behind on your clothesline for another day or so?"

"No problem. Now, Benny. If we have other kinds of visitors? If those men come back? Is it important that they stay a while?"

"Mama! Be careful. These people are real nasty. They were going to do some terrible things to Eve. Better not give them any grief."

"Would I give anyone who was bothering any of my boys any trouble? Of course not! But Benny, could you do me a favor?"

"Of course, Mama."

"Whatever else you do, please make a tiny little stop for me in Merion."

Ben made a trip to a special bin in his wine cellar before he headed down Conshohocken State Road toward Philadelphia. In Merion he stopped at Hymie's, a Jewish deli, where he completed his mission for Mama. On City Avenue Ben stopped at a pawnshop.

"Sure, we got 'em," said the man at the counter. "But who the fuck wants 'em? I'll give you a good price just to move 'em. What size?"

Ben pocketed the small envelope that held his newest purchases. He took an incredibly circuitous route to shake off possible tails before he beeped his horn in front of Lucco's house and drove by. He drove at least ten blocks away and executed an elaborate series of turns before doubling back.

Mr. Brazzo was walking an enormous Neapolitan Mastiff two blocks from his home when Ben arrived at their meeting place. They spoke in Italian. Ben handed him the envelope and a shopping bag. They killed some time discussing the Phillies' relief pitchers until both felt sure there were no interested onlookers. Ben scratched the monster dog behind his ears, and said his goodbyes. He was given a jar of Mama's red gravy, so fresh it was still hot.

FORTY-SEVEN

Lucco Brazzo came to the door of his parents' row house deep in South Philadelphia. There he found three men. All wore dark suits. All had neat haircuts. All patronized tailors whose craft had failed to conceal the less than subtle bulges beneath their jackets.

"Mr. Brazzo?"

"My Papa's Mr. Brazzo around here. You want to talk to him? I'll get him."

"No. Mr. Lucco Brazzo? Is that you?"

"And who might be inquiring?" Lucco smiled.

"Special Agent Johnson, Please don't waste our time. Are you Lucco Brazzo?"

Lucco Brazzo's smile was as genuine as Johnson's name.

"I am Lucco Brazzo. How about some identification, Mr.—uh—Johnson?"

"My orders are to not show identification unless absolutely necessary."

"Oh. So you're from some hush-hush group that works for Uncle Sam? I still would rather see some identification."

"You don't understand, Mr. Brazzo. I work for an organization that works to keep its operations secret."

"Mr. Johnson," Lucco smiled more broadly still, "Me too! I'm part of an organization that doesn't like outsiders prying in to what it does. I understand completely."

"Mr. Brazzo! Your kind of secret organization is a bunch of crooks who want to keep their fat asses out of jail! Mine upholds the law. I don't have a great sense of humor. Where is that woman? We know she's here."

"How would you know that?"

"Come on! There's an extra setting on your table every meal and the kind of underwear on your line you or your parents sure aren't wearing."

"Nice surveillance! She's out of your league, Johnson. Mine too, for that matter. Pity! Yeah. But, she's gone. Come in if you want to. Mama figured she might as well do the stuff she left with the family's laundry. Mama wants me to bring home a girl who's more like our people."

"You're wasting my time." Johnson turned to the others, who shrugged. "OK, here's my ID. You are about to be arrested for the obstruction of justice. Czisniewski! Read him his rights and frisk him."

Czisniewski Mirandized Lucco Brazzo. Minetti stood back, his hand on his weapon. Midway through patting Lucco down, Czisniewski froze.

"What? You found the mousetrap?" asked Lucco. "I said you're welcome to come in. We're law-abiding citizens. We have firearms, but they're all legal, trigger-locked, and stored safely."

Beads of sweat dotted Czisniewski's forehead. "He has strange hard objects in his jacket. Long cylinders. What do you have in there? Are those bombs?"

"No. But I really don't want you to touch them. And I don't want to take them out."

"Why not?" By now Czisniewski and Johnson had backed away. Minetti trained his weapon on Lucco.

"Minetti!" Johnson shouted, "Back off!

"Mr. Brazzo, you just admitted you're a member of a secret organization. OK, wise guy! That's cute. Yeah, I should have laughed at your little joke. But Mafia or not, you're pushing your luck. What are you packing?"

"Mr. Johnson," Lucco smiled, "May I show you something without your ape shooting me?"

"Go ahead."

Lucco slipped a ring off a thick finger and handed it to Johnson.

"Along with George Washington, Benjamin Franklin, and my own father, I am a Mason. As you know, the Masons are a secret organization. I thought it would amuse you because," and here Lucco pointed, "you three wear Masonic rings. I'm sorry. I thought you'd get the joke."

Johnson's face went blank as he returned Lucco's ring.

"And as far as what I am packing—please don't tell anyone. This could cause trouble with my Italian colleagues."

Johnson's face became animated again.

"May I? Well, you see, I am carrying contraband." Lucco reached into his jacket pockets and pulled out two small salamis.

"What kind of shit are you giving me, Brazzo? I've had enough of you."

"Mr. Johnson! Gentlemen! Please look at those salamis."

"So?"

"Look closer."

"I don't get it."

Minetti broke in. "Boss?"

"What?"

"Boss, those are Jewish salamis—Hebrew National."

Brazzo shrugged, "It's like a scandal to my mother that I prefer Hebrew National. 'That's not for you to eat,' she screams, and throws them out. So, I sneak them into the house, and I have this little refrigerator down in ..."

"You just wasted the time of—wait a minute! You held us up so that bastard Jordan had more time to get away with the girl. All this bullshit about the Masons and salami. I'll make you pay for this!"

"Mr. Johnson, if you want to find me guilty of something, I am guilty of wanting to please my father and my mother. For my father, I joined the Masons, about whom I could not care less. For my mother, I try not to upset her. I confess to being very close to my parents. Unfortunately, on this day of all days, my family connections seem to be upsetting to you. For that, I apologize. If I am free to go, I'll take my salamis and go inside. Unless you boys would like to take one along and try it later. Hebrew National. Good stuff!"

Lucco Brazzo gave Johnson, Minetti, and Czisniewski his best smile as they walked away, cursing under their breath.

"Any problems, Lucco?"

"No, Mama."

"Did they like the salami?"

"Mama, that was as good as your red gravy! Where did you get that idea?"

Lucco's father broke in. "You've got a smart Mama. You didn't get your brains from me. Just your good looks."

The two men chuckled.

"Some vino would be good, Dad."

His father produced a bottle of great Barolo.

"Since when do we drink like rich people, Dad?"

"Your friend left it with the two Masonic rings. He said that maybe later you would want to relax." He shook his head slowly. "That friend of yours, Ben?"

"Yeah, Dad?"

"What kind of man is he?"

"He doesn't pry. I don't pry. He's scary, Dad. Not 'cause he tries to scare you. He's scary because ... because when you see what he's capable of doing, and you put a few things together ... That's when you wonder, like you say, 'What kind of man is he?'"

"Has he ever done anything ...?"

"No." Lucco thought a moment. "When I start to think, I don't wonder what he could do. I wonder if there is anything he wouldn't do. You know he calls Chicago 'Uncle.'"

"Probably dangerous to think too much about that," said Mama from the kitchen.

"I think the wine has breathed enough," said Mr. Brazzo. "Mama! Please, this is worth sipping slowly."

When Mama saw the bottle, her face brightened. Then tears welled up in her eyes. She whispered something to her husband. He picked up the bottle and studied it. Soon he smiled and embraced Mama as his eyes grew moist as well.

FORTY-EIGHT

Ben left messages for three old friends, Tomasso Petrone, Rob Silverman, and Carlos Diaz. He asked Tomasso to help him acquire some information. He asked Rob to provide sanctuary for Eve if need be. He asked Carlos to find him a high performance car that looked like a piece of shit, and garage space to hide his own car for a few days.

He walked to a wooded portion of his property where two adjustable-height platforms stood about three and a half feet apart. He placed a cinder block on both platforms, and raised them until the center of each block was almost six feet off the ground. Holding his hands up and to the side, he mimicked surrender to adversaries both behind and before him. Ben whipped his arms back. Crumbling cinderblocks were still falling when he shot forward and threw a flurry of blows. Only Elani had witnessed this exercise. Ben hoped to keep it that way.

FORTY-NINE

"Ben, you OK?"

"Never better. Did the very very secret agent types like the rings?"

"Seemed to. Interesting idea."

"Yeah. When I tangled with their buddies at Eve's, I noticed they wore Masonic rings. It was worth a shot."

"Where did you get those salamis?"

"Oh! Hymie's in Merion. Your Mama's idea."

"That stuff ain't half bad, man. I might get some more. Hey! Where did you get those Masonic rings? You a Mason?"

"Sure. I was initiated into the rite of three balls at the City Line Super Pawn on the way into town. May have to freeze your Mama's red gravy."

"I won't tell her, man. She might take it personal. She thinks that spoils it."

"Shit. Thanks for reminding me. Tell her I can't use it immediately, so I'll give it to Eve to fix for the troops. You and your Dad are bad enough, but your sweet Mama—she's the scary one."

"That I'll tell her. She'll like that. And she liked your friend Eve. So much that she told me that she wished Eve was Italian.

FYI, the folks who stopped in on me were Johnson, Minetti and Czisniewski."

"Thanks for the phony names."

"Agreed. You need anything?"

"I'm thinking that Eve needs ongoing protection. Just in case those were real feds, I don't want you and your family to catch any crap. Any new ideas?"

"Nope. I'd stick with friends of friends—off duty cops."

"Still waiting on something for Eve."

"My man's on it—may take a day or so. Anything else?"

"Just cover my ass with your Mama."

"You got it. Hey, Ben?"

"That Barolo? What's with that?"

"Not to your taste?"

"No! It's great. But my Mama … She cried. My dad too, a little."

"Well, next time you're in the living room, where your Mama won't let you sit down?"

"Yeah?"

"Take a look at the smaller framed photo alongside your parents' wedding picture."

"Let me take a look. Shit! Ben! That's the same wine they drank on their honeymoon, in that café in Venice. Man. You are something! Again, Ben, you need anything?"

"Cover my ass with your Mama. Later, Lucco."

Lucco hung up the phone and sat down with his parents.

"Whatever kind of man Ben is," said Mama, "he knows something about love."

FIFTY

In deference to or fear of Mama Brazzo, Ben risked a direct run to an Italian take-out place he patronized when Elani had to be away. Once home, Ben placed the precious jar of Mama's red gravy in the apprehensive hands of Eve Gilchrist. She seemed a bit puzzled by the food he'd brought, so he gave her a brief lesson on how to serve it up, and how to rewarm the red gravy just right.

Lucco called.

"The next shift is on its way. You don't know them, but Pacella and Tomaselli vouch for them. Morales and Johnson."

"Johnson?"

"Yeah. He's a real Johnson."

"If you say so."

"The other thing, later. Second shift."

* * *

Ben showed Eve around his house.

"I have to travel. Use this tonight or Lucco's momma will destroy me. She liked you, by the way."

"That's sweet ..."

"No, you don't get it. That's a first. She hated every girl who ever came into that house, but she wishes you were Italian."

"I think she saw I liked her son. He's very smart."

"He is. And he's a good friend, but with a different sort of lifestyle. I wish I could have left you with them. They'd take a bullet rather than turn you over. But the bad guys put you under surveillance more quickly than I anticipated. The Brazzos can't risk federal investigation. You understand?"

"Like I wouldn't have understood a couple of days ago. There's a whole world I never knew existed."

"You sure I can't persuade you to spend some time with your parents?"

"I hate to admit this, but I caved. I tried to call them. They're northbound on the Intracoastal Waterway. My Dad called the embassy from a pay phone in some East Armpit, believe it or not, and told them his radio was out. He plans to put in at some big marina and replace it. The embassy contacted Washington."

"He didn't call Washington?"

"If I had to guess, my folks figured Washington would send the Coast Guard to rescue them and ruin their cruise. They're probably loving every second of their little adventure."

"You sure I can't send you to meet up with them just north of East Armpit? If I give you a travel kit with a bullhorn and Kevlar water wings? Didn't think so."

FIFTY-ONE

Ben felt obligated to talk to Jeff in person before he left town. Jeff kept him waiting till the end of the day.

Ben tolerated a series of remarks that lauded Will and implicitly showered Ben with contempt. Ben contained himself. He coaxed Jeff into granting Eve a week away from her responsibilities in the residency. Jeff offered no opposition to Ben's own request for a brief emergency leave. He seemed relieved, even pleased, that Ben would be out of his sight.

Ben read Jeff's unstated message loud and clear: *Let's see how Liebowitz pinch hits. If I fire Ben, I want to replace him with someone I won't have to worry about. Maybe I can be in California before Len starts to ask the hard questions.*

Jeff downplayed the attacks against Eve and challenged the connections Ben had drawn between those events and Joe's interview with Will.

"Your paranoia is completely over the top, Ben! You're out of touch with reality. Those incidents are regrettable. But there's no reason to connect them in some conspiracy theory."

"Eve Gilchrist's apartment was tossed! Her office was trashed! She fought off an attempt to kidnap her! Two men were torturing her to get her to tell them how to find Joe Morgan when I walked in! We ridicule conspiracy theories because usually they're fantastic and have no evidence to sustain them. But sometimes we ridicule them because we don't want to face the amazing betrayals they call to our attention. We've got a hell of a lot of evidence. That takes us from conspiracy theory to conspiracy!"

"There's no evidence. Just hunches."

"Just try to sell that conspiracy theory bullshit to Eve, or to Ambassador and Mrs. Gilchrist if things go sour. It seems to me that you're willing to sacrifice her …"

"That's it. You're fired!"

"Want to run that by the administration, Jeff? Our president is a woman. She'll be delighted to hear that you blow off attacks on …"

"I'm sorry. I just lost my temper."

"Glad you got your temper back. When your conscience shows up, let me know."

FIFTY-TWO

Jeff and Will had lunch at the Faculty Club. Will preferred its refined atmosphere and elegant fare, beyond the means of most of those its name suggested it was created to serve. Usually Will said next to nothing about his unit's research projects and evaded inquiries, but today he was talkative.

"I fault myself for this hullaballoo, Jeff. I have to apologize. I'm even partially responsible for Ben's attitude. Maybe it's more my fault than his, but don't ask me to admit that except to present company.

"I'm close-mouthed by nature. I've never really asked myself how that must appear to my colleagues, even the more rational ones. Starting now, I'll make a quarterly report to you and the faculty, and I'll keep quiet only when something needs to be kept quiet."

"That's great news, Will! If the residents see those reports and get interested, you may find you have more helping hands than you ever imagined."

"Yeah. I'm realizing that I've been a jerk! Whatever his failings, Ben brings fine young minds into the department. I've lost out by staying in my cave."

"This is music to my ears. It's a fantastic plus for the department. We may attract some residents who are research-oriented, too. We're a national powerhouse for clinical training, but there's more than that in crafting a first-rate program. You bring what it takes to make us the best."

"Thanks. It's time I really pulled my weight."

"To further the healing, let me bring you up to date on that case you worried about. There have been some surprising developments that might allay your misgivings."

"Really?"

"Eve Gilchrist's apartment was ransacked. Her office was broken into as well."

"No!"

"And she was attacked on the street. She decked the guy. Quite a gal!"

"Indeed!"

"Someone ambushed her and tried to torture her for information about this guy. Jordan happened to drop by in time to break it up, and they attacked him, too."

"That's awful! Are they OK?"

"They are. These attacks seem connected with the Joe Morgan case."

"The mystery man?"

"Yeah. Ben's come up with some external corroboration."

"Well, if that holds up, I'll need to look up some good recipes for crow—'cause I'll have a lot to eat. I hate to admit it, but if I've been wrong, I've been wrong. So, in preparation for my dubious feast, what kind of corroboration?"

"Ben traced Joe's football stories back to his real high school team."

"I owe Ben an apology, then. It sounds like he and Eve Gilchrist are doing a brilliant job. Keep me posted."

"I will. But you should know that the patient became quite aggressive with Eve Gilchrist. Ben removed her from the case for her own safety. He's going to Massachusetts to do some background research."

"I'm sure that you have things under control and you've made sure she's safe, but just for my own peace of mind, what's being done to protect that young lady? She seems like a very promising young colleague."

"Jordan has something arranged."

FIFTY-THREE

On the fourth ring, Johnson took the phone.

"Yes?"

"Our good buddy is going north to do some field work on that project."

"Fascinating. Do you think he could use some help?"

"That's a thoughtful idea."

"Maybe I'll catch up with him and offer him a hand."

"He's not expecting any help. I think he'll be incredibly grateful."

* * *

Johnson met with his direct superior. He learned that the Program was inclining toward terminating Eve Gilchrist.

"I'm surprised," said Johnson. "She really is out of the picture. May I ask how this decision was reached?"

His superior thought for a moment.

"Yes, you should be informed about the relevant considerations. Our study of Eve Gilchrist shows that she is determined, intelligent, and loyal. Her parents may be alcoholics, but they have grit.

"If we have to remove Jordan, Dr. Gilchrist herself is powerless, but her concern over Jordan, who saved her from torture, might light a fire under her father, her mother, and their families. All are very well connected and difficult to deter. Two of her uncles hold the majority of stock in a firm that provides security services to our military and government in troubled areas. It could mobilize 200 or more high-level former military operatives in less time than it takes to brew a good pot of coffee, and endanger the Program. Neither Eve Gilchrist nor her family can be intimidated. We cannot risk running afoul of her family. Jordan must go … Need I explain further?"

Neither man felt more than mild regret about ending the life of a lovely and gifted young woman. Business was business.

Johnson pondered the situation. The two operatives working with him were effective psychopaths. They would want to have their fun before they terminated the life of an extremely beautiful woman. Giving them free rein risked leaving behind a trail of evidence … To guarantee maximal protection to the Program, he would have to kill Eve himself.

He equipped himself with a .22 revolver, paired it with a powerful suppressor, and selected ammunition with enough power to penetrate a victim's skull, but not enough to forge an exit through bone. His slugs would destroy Eve's brain as they ricocheted inside her skull.

FIFTY-FOUR

Ben checked on Eve one more time. He assigned her a paper to write over the next few days, minimizing the risk she'd lose credit for time in training if Jeff had a change of heart.

He chatted with the day shift and met Tony Pacella, who'd just arrived. The next shift, Pacella and Frank Tomaselli, were Lucco's boyhood friends.

"Pacella is an old-fashioned family man," Lucco told Ben. "His buddy, Tomaselli, still chases skirts. But when he's on duty, he's on duty. They're solid cops."

Ben reviewed the situation and said goodbyes all around. Time to go. He picked up Conshohocken State Road and jumped onto 476 North at Conshohocken. From 476 he switched onto the Pennsylvania Turnpike, 276 East toward New Jersey, then north up the New Jersey Turnpike toward Rob Silverman's home.

He tried to focus on Joe Morgan, but events at the U kept intruding. *I could be out of a job by the time I get back.*

FIFTY-FIVE

On a private beach near Netanya, in Israel, three old friends laughed, talked, and kept the white wine flowing. Elani Weisenthal Jordan was enjoying the company of old friends, Rakel Nusbaum and Danielle Stern. Tanning topless on the secluded estate of Danielle's rich American relatives, they felt completely secure. After an iced bottle of pino grigio and a couple hours of breezy conversation, they uncorked a second and were sliding into a silly mood.

Two men wearing jackets and ties despite the scorching heat and the informality Israelis favored drew quite near before they were noticed. The women reached for their wraps in a flurry of motion.

"Elani Jordan?"

Danielle stood and stared the men down.

"This is private property. Get out! Get out now!"

The second man unfolded a piece of paper. He scrutinized it carefully, and pointed at Elani. "The tallest one."

The first man spoke again.

"Mrs. Jordan, you have to come with us. Now."

"Credentials?" Elani asked.

Both men reached inside their jackets. Before either could draw, Elani kicked one in the crotch and broke the other man's nose. Rakel placed the first in a chokehold, while Danielle knocked down the second. Elani confiscated their weapons.

"Strip!" Elani commanded.

"Fuck you!"

Elani shot twice into the sand, barely missing the speaker's shoes, and handed one gun to Rakel.

"Danielle, this is your family's place. Why don't you call the police?"

"You can't do that!" the first man screamed.

"What did you say to me before that?" Elani asked.

There was silence. Elani's bullet missed the man's foot by millimeters.

"I said, 'Fuck you!'"

"Then you know my response. Hey, Danielle?"

"What?"

"Forget the police. Call Mossad."

Both shed most of their clothing as quickly as they could.

"Don't stop. Everything. Face down on the sand, hands behind your backs."

"You can't ..."

"I can. Two armed foreigners trespassing on private property, and attempting to kidnap an Israeli woman ... That may interest the authorities."

"But ..."

"My next shot will deliver a stronger message. If you must relieve yourselves, do so without moving. Lie still and silent. Enjoy the sun. Get a nice tan, and make up happy little stories to tell your friendly colleagues in the local police and Mossad."

FIFTY-SIX

The new arrival, Lieutenant Tony Pacella, was a pleasant, balding, somewhat overweight man in a rumpled suit. He carried a slim gun case. After Ben left, he took a chair near Eve.

"I'm part of your next shift. Lieutenant Tony Pacella, Philadelphia PD. I'm a licensed gun dealer and registered gun collector. Back in high school, a couple dozen pounds ago, I played football with a big friend of yours who sends his regards. His movements are … currently restricted."

"Is he OK?"

"Yes. He asked me to ask you to come up with some story to explain why I might have stopped in with this thing."

"You mean about how I met you at a gun show I stumbled into when I was antiquing out in Lancaster County, Amish country? I remember your smiling face and that I beat you on the price, but I don't remember your name."

Pacella smiled and handed her the case and a box of cartridges.

"That works. Is this what you had in mind? It's a Beretta side by side. Youth model. Your friend described you as, uh, very slender in frame. With the shorter barrel, it's better for inside work. Better small than oversized when you gotta be quick at close quarters. More recoil than I'd like for you, but there wasn't much time to pick and choose."

Eve inspected the gun, and threw it to her shoulder. She put it down, grabbed it, brought it to hip level, and swept the weapon around.

"No civilian taught you that."

No, Uncle Buck was no civilian! Eve nodded.

"Adequate?"

Eve nodded again. "Solo?" she asked.

"No."

"Help's right outside?"

"Check it out."

"Where?"

"Your friend had a feeling. He asked us to cruise the neighborhood when we arrived."

"Where is your car?"

"Nowhere nearby. Frank Tomaselli is looking around. He'll be here in a minute if we need him."

"How will he know?"

"Say hello, Frank."

"Hello," came a voice from Tony Pacella's neck. "Wired, Dr. Gilchrist. Wired. Tony, I'm going to check this place out. I'll be quick. A black Blazer was cruising by real slow near here on Conshohocken. Three guys. Not too subtle. Thought I saw a gun barrel. Not even trying to cover up. They're either complete assholes or they know something we don't know."

"Roger."

A few minutes later Frank Tomaselli made his appearance. A lanky, casually dressed man in his forties, he stood half a foot taller than Pacella. His cynical sneer seemed to be the natural state of his face. When Tomaselli actually saw Eve, he did a double take. Then Pacella caught his eye, and he calmed down.

"Eve," said Tony, "This is Frank Tomaselli. He was the star of our team.

"He's not quite as nasty as he looks."

"Philadelphia's least eligible bachelor," Frank joked. "Pleased to meet you, Dr. Gilchrist."

"Cover things, Frank." Pacella left to recheck the house and the grounds. When he returned, the two reversed roles and repeated their sweep.

When they both sat down with Eve, Frank reported seeing the three men in a Blazer. Eve told them about the men in the blue Blazer in South Philly. The policemen exchanged a meaningful glance.

Tomaselli went into another room and called the Lower Merion PD. He returned looking puzzled.

"Shift commander took the call personally. Earlier today three navy cops walked into the station. Said they were an NIS team following up on reports of violence by one Joseph Morgan, a former Marine. Said they'd checked in at Gladwyne already. They've been driving by the Gilchrist and Jordan residences trying to intercept him. Said they'd be coming here to offer Dr. Gilchrist protective custody if they can't catch up to this Morgan fella. Their ride is a black Blazer."

Eve excused herself. She checked her home message machine. It was empty. She started to check her office machine, then remembered it had been destroyed.

"I can't be sure whether or not they left me a message," she explained.

"If they show up, Dr. Gilchrist," Pacella asked, "How do you want to play it?"

"I just don't know. I'm confused beyond confusion."

* * *

Eve set about preparing a late dinner. Pacella and Tomaselli pitched in, one at a time, the second remaining on alert and periodically checking the grounds. Both knew the place where Ben got the food, and loved Mama's red gravy.

While Eve and Tomaselli ate at the table, Pacella took his plate and a chair to a window overlooking the driveway. Every few minutes Tomaselli rose, and checked out the illuminated back yard area. With dinner came conversation. Pacella alternately boasted and worried aloud about his brood of children, especially his "bright and gorgeous" oldest daughter.

Tomaselli told a series of hilarious but painful stories about his athletic career and failed marriages. Eve shared some of her sillier escapades from times when she knew no better.

After a while, a vehicle drove slowly up Ben's driveway. A man walked toward the house, wearing a big smile and waving a white handkerchief.

"Sorry if I surprised you folks," said Czisniewski. "Norman Johnson, NIS, Northeast Regional Office. I figured you probably wouldn't answer your phone, but I didn't know a better way to say hello without … You know …" He shrugged, and smiled.

"Yeah," said Pacella. "We heard you were in this neck of the woods."

"You guys are sharp. Was that one of you in the station wagon giving us the evil eye a few minutes back?"

"Guilty," Tomaselli confessed.

"Let me show you my credentials and orders, and bring my men out of the cold. Goldman! Come on in. Michaels, take the ride and sweep the surveillance locations once more, just in case. Then gas up and get back here."

Minetti, now a.k.a. Goldman, put on his friendliest grin, waved, and came up to the house. Johnson a.k.a. Michaels waved from the Blazer and drove off. Pacella and Tomaselli studied their papers.

"Why NIS?"

Czisniewski a.k.a. Johnson laughed.

"Good question. Dr. Gilchrist seems to be in some danger from a former marine who may have experienced some messing with his mind, maybe brainwashing. Marine or naval personnel plus anything connected to intelligence or terrorism, that's us. Also, we have safe houses that may be useful resources.

"Believe it or not, NIS has several big regional offices and many smaller substations throughout the US. Northeast goes from Maine to Pennsylvania. We're from the big office in Newport, Rhode Island. NIS couldn't spring a team from one of the closer offices—staffing's too thin. We have the honor of being the least necessary three agents in Newport, or maybe the ones who pissed off the station chief most recently. Yeah—check option number two."

Everyone chuckled. Tomaselli nodded, "Been there! Been there!"

"Look. If it's OK with you, we'll grab something to eat and come back, pick up Dr. Gilchrist, and head north." He handed them his papers again. "Feel free to check us out. I would if I were you. That stuff smells great. Did you get it around here?"

Pacella and Tomaselli exchanged glances, nodded.

"Pitch in, boys. There's more than enough," said Pacella.

After a few bites, Czisniewski/Johnson exclaimed, "Oh, man! I gotta piss off the chief again, real soon!"

Tomaselli called the numbers on the documents. Everyone he reached vouched for Norman Johnson and his team. A man identified as a senior NIS official ended his confirmation by telling Tomaselli that he wanted to talk to Johnson and communicate a change in orders. "Listen in. Put it on speaker. It's nothing secret. Johnson, you're in a safe, defensible place. It's late. Your team is exhausted. Stay where you are tonight. Make your return run tomorrow morning."

"OK," said Czisniewski/Johnson, "We'll crash here tonight. When Michaels gets back, we'll bring in sleeping bags. We won't mess up the place."

He turned to Pacella and Tomaselli. "Might as well call off the next shift. NIS will stand watch."

Pacella and Tomaselli exchanged glances. Pacella turned to Eve.

"Dr. Gilchrist, how does this sit with you? We're willing to stay."

Eve's mind was reeling. *So Ben isn't the only one who's afraid I'm in danger! If an agency like NIS is getting involved, I really better take this seriously. And I hate to be an imposition.* Balancing her wish not to be a burden against her reluctance to be under government protection, she sighed, and agreed to accept the NIS offer.

They continued to eat and talk until the Philly cops left. Even though the NIS men were quite respectful, Eve felt uncomfortable with them.

FIFTY-SEVEN

When Johnson reached Junior, they bantered about work and women, decided it was too late to have a few beers, and said goodnight.

In fact, Junior would be on duty until the mission in Gladwyne was completed, monitoring his taps and redirecting mission-critical calls to or from Ben Jordan's home. After Johnson learned Pacella and Tomaselli had left, he drove back to Gladwyne. Eve had shown she would spit in the face of harsh interrogation, so Johnson planned to present himself as a kind helper. He'd gamble that if he and his entire team remained courteous and friendly, Eve might simply tell him what he needed to know before he brought her life to the tragic and premature conclusion the Program had ordained.

FIFTY-EIGHT

Eve Gilchrist worked to present herself as a poised and somewhat aloof ice princess. If pressed, she would admit that Elani, her current ideal, was a fallback icon. Eve really wanted to be like Grace Kelly, and regretted having become too voluptuous to imitate her appearance. Both her warmth and her eye-catching attributes defeated her efforts to affect a glacial pulchritude. Men tended to see her more as an object of desire than the thing of perfect untouchable beauty she aspired to be.

Eve was exquisitely uncomfortable. Superficial courtesy notwithstanding, three of the four men couldn't take their eyes off of her. When Tomaselli left, she thought her discomfort would diminish. Instead, it skyrocketed. As evening passed into night, Eve suffered the first true panic attacks of her life.

Panic is weakness! That's something patients have! Eve was mortified to be overtaken by emotions she considered beneath her. Terror soared to a level beyond her imagination. Soon it owned Eve Gilchrist.

She remembered Ben's first observations—she was afraid of her feelings. Jeff and Ben had talked to her about how important it was for therapists to use their reactions to their patients, normal or abnormal, good or bad, acceptable or loathsome, as valuable sources of information.

Since Pacella and Tomaselli left, I don't feel safe.

But why are they making me more nervous? Tomaselli was undressing me with his eyes all evening. What makes it worse now? These two are supposed to be the squeaky clean Feds.

But they were the ones who really made her nervous! No matter how she tried to think through her situation, Eve got nowhere.

What would Ben do? That's a sad joke for a girl raised to think, "What would Jesus do?" One notion after another floated through her mind, all things she was sure Ben wouldn't do.

And then it came to her. *As usual, I'm trying to* figure *out what I might do wrong and get in trouble, and trying to avoid doing it. That's how I've been since I got my act together. Ben would use his emotions as information. He would grind along in that ruthless problem-solving mode of his. That's what Ben would do!*

When she gave herself permission to censor her own censorship, Eve discovered feelings she considered disgusting and usually blocked out at once. *I'm upset. All these men with their eyes glued on me.* From the time her developing body demonstrated its power to captivate male attention, Eve had schooled herself to ignore being checked out by dozens to hundreds of men every day. Suppose she let herself be less glacial? What could she learn about the men who were unsettling her?

From what Eve considered a cruder and coarser female perspective on the men she had to deal with, Ray, whom she knew would arrive soon, was a mildly interesting man with some simple straightforward virtues and charms. But he was boringly good. He was brilliant, but rarely let it show. Sadly, Ray was damaged goods, more driven to staunch his own emotional hemorrhaging than drawn to engage with others. His deep dark puppy dog eyes would be attractive, if they weren't misting over with sadness from time to time. Ray seemed a bit intimidated by her. He was not comfortable with A-list people. She hated herself for thinking, *A mercy fuck at best.*

Goldman a.k.a. Minetti crossed her mind next. A cold fish! Yes, he had appraised her, and seemed to want her, but his wanting seemed without passion or desire, more a matter of control and domination. To him she was a pretty thing that happened to be a woman. *He would take me if he could, just because he could.* He evoked no positive reactions or empathic connection at all. *He could kill me without a qualm!*

Johnson a.k.a. Czisniewski was a letch. He made no attempts to relate. He just salivated from afar. *He wants to fuck me just to say he did it. He might even want to hurt me. But in a million years, he would never make love to me. Could he even sustain a relationship with a woman?*

Tomaselli seemed infatuated, but he understood she was hands off and behaved accordingly. She found Pacella attractive in a funny way. As they had talked he had become delighted with her as a person. Over and over again he talked about his daughter Maria, and told Eve that he hoped his own daughter would grow up to be like her. Eve found herself promising to talk to Maria about medical careers. Their conversations had been warm and loving, about relationships among fathers and mothers and daughters. If she could adopt Pacella into her own family, she would make it so in a heartbeat.

Lucco surprised her. The big man was clearly a thug, but he was brilliant and thoughtful. His self-education was truly impressive. To her amusement and amazement, despite his complete lack of conventional good looks, Lucco Brazzo turned her on. They were too different to work together, but the electricity was powerful.

She hadn't really met the man who'd stayed in the car, but his men scared her. Could he be more terrifying still?

Then there was Ben. The more she saw of him, the more she appreciated him. She had never considered dating an older man, but she found herself wondering. But Ben clearly was completely in love with his wife, a woman Eve knew only from her striking appearance on magazine covers. He treated his pretty resident as if she were a daughter.

But what could she actually expect? Ruthlessly, she considered that since she was a beautiful woman, she might have fallen into the trap of focusing on what was readily accessible once she stopped running from it. *But how to look deeper …*

Her eye fell upon one of Ben's yellow Levenger pads, the kind he used when he'd tracked her dynamics with unsettling accuracy. Eve told Ben he was dangerous. He had replied that it was his job to make her dangerous, too. She'd read the Luborsky book. *Have I learned enough?*

Eve grabbed the pad and the gold Cross ballpoint she used almost every day to do the *New York Times* crossword puzzle. *Ben uses a pencil. He takes a while to be sure. Me, I'm too sure too fast.* She put down her gold ballpoint and dug out her rarely used Pentel Quicker-Clicker pencil. *What am I becoming?*

Eve set up a separate page for each man in the house: Tomaselli, Pacella, Johnson (Czisniewski), and Goldman (Minetti). She made columns for the CCRT components: subject, what is desired, the object from whom it is desired, and inner and outer factors that impede or help the subject in getting what the subject wants in life.

Then she made a second sheet for each man and tried to write down everything she remembered about everything he talked about, dividing what she remembered into incidents. That took her well over an hour. Ben had told her that Luborsky's group hadn't concluded how many incidents needed to be analyzed, but perhaps ten or twelve might do the job. No way she would have that many! She would do the best she could.

Pacella probably would be the easiest. She looked at her notes.

"You hung in there, Eve, all those years. Now, look at you! I hope Maria sticks to her dreams. She wants to be a vet, but she'll settle for being a people doc. I just don't know how to encourage her, you know, to stay the course. It's hard. Like you, she's pretty. The boys … Ah, you know! I mean, I always wanted to be a cop. I kept my nose clean, kept in shape, and here I am. But that was easy in comparison."

Eve was not sure she was on the right track, but for subject, she wrote "I." For wish, she guessed "Maria's dreams." For object, she wrote "Maria." For facilitating the goal, she wrote, "staying the course." For problematic obstructions, she wrote "long time" and "boys."

How does that look? Eve asked herself. If that holds true, a formulation might turn out to be, "I want to help my daughter Maria to fulfill her dreams, but can she stay the course? I am afraid the prospect of long years of study and her interest in boys may sabotage her dreams and my dreams for her, and I feel helpless to protect her." She knew that was too complex and wordy, but she felt she was getting the gist of it. She scored four more vignettes, and was stunned by their consistency. Pacella had either been talking about Maria or herself, but his total preoccupation was with the well-being of young women, and at four to one, Maria, not Eve, stayed in the formulation.

Next, she worked up Tomaselli. Tomaselli seemed to talk about things he desired but could not have. Whether he talked about a sports car, a dream vacation, or something else, which Eve thought might be a displacement from his interest in her in the moment, it was almost the same thing. The gist was consistent. After seven brief vignettes, Tomaselli's story seemed to be: "I want [so many things] from [so many people] but I am way past my chance to get them, and [a range of people] don't want me to have what I want." Just like her gut instincts! Tomaselli desired her, but knew that she was off limits and that even if she were not, she was unlikely to respond to any older man, especially not to him. *If he were my patient*, Eve thought, *I never would have suspected such disappointment and sadness!*

Now, Goldman (Minetti) had a usually Jewish name, but didn't seem Jewish at all. He had said relatively little, but from the perspective of the raw CCRT data, Eve felt a chill sweep over her as his columns filled.

He had said, to no one in particular, "What we need to do is clean up this mess. And do it right, and right away. No loose ends. Excuse me, Dr. Gilchrist. I need to get that envelope under your pocketbook. We're wasting time." Cryptic, requiring inference, but telling. The other three episodes were fragmentary, and couldn't be scored completely. In desperation, Eve threw them into the mix.

She came up with: "I want to get rid of everything/everyone in my way but I can't do that yet because ..." The clear inference was that this man was waiting for orders or permission to deal with what disturbed him. That might mean her!

That left Johnson (Czisniewski). He favored war stories. In every one, he was pissed at someone, and that someone no longer was around to bother him. *This man would shoot me and fuck me as I died, smiling all the way*, Eve wrote.

Am I blowing this out of proportion? Can I really make decisions based on stuff like this? As she pondered, she found herself removing the Beretta from its case, and loading both chambers. She wished it were an automatic. At some deeper level, she knew the answer.

She snapped the weapon closed, ready to fire. Too noisy! She reached under the couch and readied the Glock. Ben had insisted she keep it on hand until help arrived. *Some help!*

She willed herself into stillness and silence.

Sitting in the next room, Czisniewski and Minetti were growing tired and irritable. Minetti was trying to get Czisniewski to keep his voice down.

"Who the fuck cares? She's got to be asleep by now. A real shame to waste such a sweet piece of ass."

This was all too real. Ben was on his way to Massachusetts. Could she call Lucco Brazzo? Eve reached out for the telephone. Too late she realized her hands were shaking.

The phone clattered to the floor.

"Shit! She's awake!"

Eve threw an afghan over the weapons.

Minetti stuck his head into the room. He raced to grab the yellow sheets of paper before Eve could gather them up.

"That's confidential research information …"

Minetti read rapidly. "Pacella? You got him right. Tomaselli? Yeah, he's pathetic!"

Then he paused. "Me? Right on target. Hah! You nailed Czis—uh, Johnson pretty good. I've seen him do that. Well, Missy, I guess we better keep a closer eye on you. I've got some cuffs here. I won't put them on too tight. Damn, this stuff about my buddy is fantastic.

"Pretty clever stuff, Dr. G." As he looked up from the papers he froze, at first unable to register and make sense of what he saw. It took him a few seconds before he could make himself believe his own eyes.

FIFTY-NINE

"Well, Ben! The kids are OK. We were sunbathing when these two men in suits and ties showed up on the beach, looking for me. We dealt with them and Mossad took them into custody. A friend promised to fill me in when they learn what's going on. Love you."

Ben felt a quick surge of panic. Will's implacable hostility, the attacks on Eve—and now this message!

Are those bastards going after Elani to get me off the case? To force me to give them information they think I have?

He tried every number he knew to reach Elani. For all intents and purposes, she was off the grid. Finally he called Rakel's husband, Yossi.

"Hello, fellow bachelor Ben!"

"Hello, fellow bachelor Yossi! I need to ask you a favor."

"Ask, my friend."

"I guess it was earlier today, or maybe yesterday, two bastards approached the girls. They were after Elani. Apparently the girls kicked ass and Mossad took them into custody."

"Yeah! I heard. I assumed Elani told you. I got to tell you, Ben, I was upset. They treated it like a big joke. Like they always do."

"You read my mind! Look, some weird stuff is happening here. I'm really worried. Please let the girls know I think they should be on the alert for more of the same."

"I know where to find them. Pray for them, and pray for me to survive Israeli traffic on the way. I think I will bring them some presents. Old, but serviceable."

"Like both of us. I'll start with the Sh'ma Yisroel ..."

"And I'll start with the Uzis and some Czech goodies. Amen and Amen."

SIXTY

Minetti shook his head in disbelief. The little Barbie Doll with all her rings and things was on her feet, holding a shotgun pointed down and away. Her finger rested gently on the trigger guard.

"That's not what they teach you in gun safety courses, Missy. Crack that thing."

Eve stood silent, immobile.

"Enough of this bullshit, already. Just give me the damn gun before you hurt yourself. I don't think you even know how to use it. Just hand it over. Hey! You don't think you know how to shoot that thing, do you? You ever shot somebody? Killed somebody? This is a joke. Right?"

Eve stood silent. Did she know how to shoot that thing? *Uncle Buck taught me well! And then all that skeet shooting and hunting with Mom and Dad!* But to raise a weapon against another human being was different. *Can I really do this?*

Her silence enraged Minetti.

"Well?"

"Yes and No."

"Don't fuck with me. 'Yes' to what? 'No' to what?"

"That's your problem."

"OK, enough smart-ass shit! If I had the time I could teach a stuck-up bitch like you a lesson you'd never forget. Hell! You might like it."

He took a step forward, his face darkening with fury.

"Hand it over. Little girl, you don't know how to shoot that thing! You'll just knock yourself on your ass. Let me tell you how it is. You hand that over or things are going to get real serious. Not very good for you! Cooperate, or we'll take it out on you. Pretty girl like you, it'll be up close and personal. We'll let my buddy do what he does. Give me the gun."

"Big man," Eve hardly recognized her own voice. Was she watching herself, hearing herself? Somehow she'd reached down deep for something she never knew was there.

"Big man, did you ever face down a rich bitch taught to shoot by Marines? Let me tell you how it is." As she spoke, she swung the Beretta toward Minetti.

"If I can knock a clay pigeon out of the sky nine times out of ten, do you really think I'll miss your fat ass a couple yards away?"

"Watch out behind you, bitch!" He reached back for his automatic.

Eve fired before she turned, just as she'd practiced. *No one behind me!* She wheeled back to see Czisniewski charging toward her, fumbling with his shoulder holster. Eve fired point-blank into his chest, dropped to the floor, rolled to cover behind a couch, and reloaded.

Only then did she look toward Minetti. His chest and abdomen were destroyed. He had collapsed, his face locked for all eternity in unspoken astonishment and horror.

Beyond Minetti, Czisniewski lay broken, his pellet-savaged body folded over the top of a big beige sofa that was beginning to turn very, very red. Eve thanked heaven that she couldn't see his face.

She braced herself for whatever might happen next. *If I weren't terrified, I wouldn't even touch that damn Purdey. I could buy a Mercedes or a Jag for less. But for all I know, the third one is coming.*

She took a deep breath, and loaded the Purdey. She chambered a round in the Glock, and placed it carefully at her side.

Then, only then, was there time to shiver, to shake, and to vomit over and over and over. Tears began to flow. From somewhere came the thought, *If only Uncle Buck were here!* She wept and fidgeted with a handful of tissues. *Even Ben. But he would just say, "That's Eve—she killed two men and barfed all over the place, but not a drop, not a single drop, landed on those designer clothes." But if Uncle Buck or Ben were here, maybe my heart would stop beating so wildly that it seems to want to jump out of my chest and leap out the nearest door or window.*

SIXTY-ONE

Johnson, dressed in black, parked the team's Blazer down Ben's driveway and began to load his suppressed .22. One blast and then another shattered the still darkness. Johnson felt a rare surge of panic. *I've got two good men in there! Something's gone very wrong!* He moved toward Jordan's house as quietly as his worries allowed.

* * *

Ray Hawkes rolled out of bed, flattening himself on the floor. In seconds, cold sweat drenched his body. *Where am I? Where the hell am I?* In a fraction of a second that lasted forever he realized that his fingernails were digging into the deep pile of a plush carpet, not the mud of Southeast Asia. He held his fingers to his nose to be sure. Then there was a second blast.

Ray had just returned from a visit with Douglas Blake. For several glorious days they fished for largemouth bass in the morning, worked on a paper in the afternoon, and sipped bourbon and shot the breeze with Blake's family as evening fell. He had picked up a message that Ben got a late start heading north. He arrived at Ben's coach house later than expected, unpacked, and crashed. *But what the hell was happening now?*

The gunshots came from Ben's house. *Was Ben back already? No way. He'd be no further than New Haven if he took 95. Elani was in Israel. But Eve was at Ben's.* Ray slipped into dark sweats and well-worn moccasins. Finding nothing that looked like a weapon, he grabbed a heavy flashlight.

Running lightly on the outside edges of his soles, Ray suppressed his footfalls as best he could. He made out sounds of another person running closer to the house, someone who was very quiet for a white man.

* * *

Johnson flattened himself against the front wall of Ben's house, alongside a picture window. Using a miniature periscope, slender enough to be overlooked at point blank range, he moved from window to window, surveying the interior rooms.

Through a side window Johnson made out the form of a slender woman. She wept and shook as she knelt on the floor, clinging to a shotgun. *Gilchrist?* Every few seconds she wiped away her tears, looked around with a stunned and terrified expression, and began to weep again. Johnson struggled to grasp that the body folded over the couch surrounded by a large red stain and the crumpled bloody heap on the floor had to be Minetti and Czisniewski.

* * *

Raymond T. Hawkes, M.D., born Ramon Two Hawks, melted into the night, moving almost silently through the darkness. He heard movement as he neared the house, and spied a figure briefly outlined against a window, holding a handgun with an unusually long barrel. The figure scuttled from window to window, finally crouching alongside one.

One hand affixed what seemed to be a suction device to a windowpane. A second dragged a small instrument around its margins. The glass was removed without a sound. The figure reached in, and unlatched the window's lock.

The figure was vulnerable with both hands occupied and the gun holstered while it opened the window. But Ray was too far away to race in. Charging an armed man who has to reach down, draw his pistol, and fire is risky, but the charging man has a good chance if he's fast and has less than fourteen or fifteen feet to cover. But Ray was behind a tree forty feet away and no sprinter. Charging would be suicidal.

Ray knew Ben's house, but not what was happening inside. Making his way to the open window, Ray heard the crash of overturning furniture and a woman's scream. He waited for another sound to screen his entry. When the woman screamed, "I can't move! You're hurting me!" Ray slipped in.

* * *

Eve had heard a soft sound. Suddenly the couch and Czisniewski's body tumbled over on top of her. Shaking her head clear, Eve found herself pinned to the floor by an overturned couch. Czisniewski's glassy-eyed death mask loomed above her. The Beretta she'd clung to with all her might was crushed against her chest—she couldn't wrench it free.

Someone had crept up behind the couch where Czisniewski had collapsed and tipped it over on her. Before Eve could get free, someone punched the side of her head and pulled her necklace. When it broke apart someone grabbed her by her hair and dragged her out just far enough to control her arms one at a time. She felt one wrist being cuffed, and then the other. A man dragged her from under the couch by her cuffed hands and shoved her back against it. Holding her arms above her head with one hand, he slapped her hard with the other, open palm and backhand, over and over.

"What the fuck did you do to Czisniewski and Minetti? You killed my men, bitch!"

Ray heard the man's anger, the harsh slaps, and Eve's whimpers rising into a wail. He crept noiselessly toward a back staircase. Ascending the carpeted steps without a sound, he crawled the length of an upper hall, and made his way down a different stairway.

Somewhere in Johnson's mind he knew he should control his feelings and cuff Eve more effectively, hands behind her back. But his rage and his certainty he would kill her within minutes betrayed him. "You've got a lot of explaining to do, bitch! Where's that motherfucker Jordan?" Another slap! Johnson threw Eve's Beretta across the room.

"You killed two federal agents, bitch! Two agents in the line of duty! Anyone who carries a badge would drop everything to take down a cop-killer. For the first time in your stuck-up fancy-ass, rich-bitch life, more men'd like to kill you than fuck you. Now, talk!"

Johnson drew back his right arm to slap Eve again. She began to beg, "No! No! No!" Then her eyes darted past him. Johnson turned just in time for Ray's fist to break his nose, just in time for Ray's mag-light swing to land a hammer blow to the side of his head and knock him to the ground.

Johnson rolled away. As Ray leaped after him, Johnson kicked the couch toward him. It rolled back onto Eve, who screamed in pain. Ray turned toward Eve. She lay among several weapons, half-covered by the couch! His pause gave Johnson time to draw his .22 and fire. Eve heard two cough-like sounds. Ray staggered and fell, struck in his right thigh and left shoulder. Johnson rolled further, scrambled to his feet, and dove through the open window.

Why is he running? Ray's attacker had missed his chance to grab a more potent weapon from either Eve or the fallen men. *With just the .22, no way he'd stay to face the Glock and shotguns!*

He turned to tell Eve they would be OK. *Where is she?* He heard light footsteps racing away. Eve and the Purdey were gone.

Eve didn't see the Beretta Johnson threw aside. She grabbed the Purdey and rocketed out of the house. *If you try to escape, you bastard, you'll go for your ride.*

There he was! The man who slapped her around and broke her necklace moved almost silently, bent low to the ground. *Like a clay pigeon skittering down, almost too low to hit.* There was no way Eve could hold and shoot normally while handcuffed, but nothing would stop her from taking her shot.

Eve brought the Purdey up with a clumsy pistol grip, let loose, and ducked as the shotgun jumped, its uncontrolled barrels nearly hitting her face. Once more Eve aimed and fired. The leaping shotgun's barrels grazing her cheek.

"Shit!" Her target seemed more surprised than enraged. Johnson paused briefly and reached behind himself. He felt the blood, cursed, and limped off as best he could. Eve cracked the Purdey to reload only to realize that she'd run after her assailant without extra shells. Johnson staggered to the black Blazer, and sped off.

Ray hobbled over to where Eve stood.

"At least I shot the bastard in the ass," said Eve.

"Nice to have a happy ending."

"I thought only Ben said such stupid shit. Before I get all up-tight and proper," Eve stood on tiptoes and kissed Ray on the cheek, "thanks for saving my life."

* * *

In an ambulance en route to the Bryn Mawr Hospital, Ray marveled at the ruthless objectivity of the thoughts racing through his mind. *Shot twice and not stopped? Not even knocked down? No real blast when the son of a bitch fired? Small caliber suppressed fire! That bastard came to do a hit on Eve! He never thought he'd need real stopping power, a heavier slug. He couldn't count on bringing me down unless he got a perfect kill shot or blasted a knee. When he couldn't grab something heavier quick, he had to make tracks. He knew he'd be outgunned in seconds.*

This evil man was trying to kill Eve Gilchrist. Ray was gripped with a sense of outrage more powerful than he had ever known. Before he reached the emergency ward, he'd sworn an oath to a God in whom he barely believed to become a *ga'an*, a protective spirit, for a woman he hardly knew, and to watch over her until she was safe from danger.

SIXTY-TWO

Ben retrieved messages from a service center payphone on the New Jersey Turnpike. He reached Ray at the Bryn Mawr Hospital.

"Ray, I'm so sorry. How are you doing?"

"Took worse in 'Nam once upon a time."

"How is Eve?"

"Unbelievably tough little gal. She got up, handcuffs and all, and shot him in the ass on the way out."

"So we should look for a bastard with a broken nose who can't sit down?"

"You got it."

"We need to get you both under protection."

"The local cops don't seem to want to do any more than drive by from time to time."

"I have something different in mind. I really don't think they know you from Adam so I doubt you're in long term danger. But just to be sure I recommend that when you're discharged, go to a hotel till this blows over. I'm coming back to pick up a few things. You won't see me. But I have to take Eve someplace safe. Someone will bring you home from the hospital."

Before Ray could tell Ben that he could take care of himself, that he couldn't afford a hotel, and that he already had studied the Joe Morgan materials, Ben was gone.

SIXTY-THREE

Ben's ruthless reasoning prevailed over his machismo. He knew he was too upset to drive further. At the next exit he took a room in a motel.

When he reached Gladwyne the next morning, Pacella and Demchak were guarding Eve. After they reviewed the recent events, Ben inspected the damage. He made a series of apologetic calls to his friends and the people he had planned to visit in New England, changing arrangements and rescheduling appointments. But one additional call now became all-important.

* * *

At first Tomasso Petrone didn't recognize the ring tone of his red phone. It had never rung before. He instructed his secretary to hold all calls and inform his next appointment he might be a few minutes late.

"Ben? The coast is clear."

"Tomasso, I need some help."

"Ask." Tomasso braced himself.

"Still tight with Stover?"

"Sure."

"Is he still on the House Permanent Select Committee on Intelligence?"

"Sure. It looks good to have an ex-SEAL on board."

"I have a problem. What I need to know is whether some really nasty people are really and officially ours."

"That's pretty high level stuff. Why do you need to know?"

"I'd just like to know who may be trying to kill me, and whom I may have to kill."

"Shit!"

Ben told Tomasso all he knew.

"This may take a while."

"Understood. Got any place I can park someone?"

"My kids are squatting every place, partying with friends."

"I can't bring this closer to your family. I'll find another way."

His next calls were to contractors. Building contractors.

SIXTY-FOUR

Ben and Pacella were nailing a large sheet of plywood over the destroyed window when Ben's hot pink phone rang. "If you and Tomasso wanted to play James Bond games," Elani had decreed, "I reserve veto power in matters of décor!"

"Stover wants to talk to you. He's on the line. You guys want me to get lost?"

Representative Elias Stover, former Navy SEAL, Baptist minister, and sitting congressman from an urban district in Detroit, relished using the rhetoric of the pulpit in everyday conversation. Its absence was ominous.

"Stick around, Tomasso. This trouble may come your way. Ben, you've run into real bad boys. This so-called Johnson is Frederick Moore. He ran a CIA project for developing very specialized field agents. They defunded his project, and he went rogue. He hijacked some very precious human experiments, men in training to become some kind of super-couriers, super-assassins. We couldn't bring them back in. They've all gone off the grid, presumably with him. There are rumors that his project is continuing, funded by a very well-disguised and well-protected foundation that influences a number of senators."

"OK, Stove," said Tomasso, "but to what end?"

"Bottom line: There are always people who feel they would be better off if someone else got taken out of the picture, people willing to pay top dollar to improve their quality of life as they see it."

"So these are freelance assassins?" Ben asked.

"Worse." Stover sighed again. Then there was another sigh. He continued, "You want to get rid of a dictator, they're freelance freedom fighters. You want to get rid of people who want to take down a dictator, they're freelance fascists. You want to get rid of people different from you, they're freelance terrorists or ethnic cleansers. You want to exchange the old model for a real model, a trophy wife, and they're freelance murderers or very inexpensive divorce lawyers."

"Are you shitting me?" Ben and Tomasso spoke at once.

"I wish I were. They cover their tracks effectively and they're not fond of leaving witnesses."

"What would they want with a student at the U?"

"The U has a few contracts with that foundation."

"Anything more?"

"Not that I can share. Steer clear."

"Too late."

"Then you may want to involve the authorities. You know how to protect yourself, but you have to be concerned about keeping these other people safe. Moore's core group was American, but we've heard he's brought people on board from all over the globe. I wish I could offer you more."

There was a long silence. Then Ben spoke.

"Stove, my home has been invaded. They tortured and tried to kill one of my students. They shot a good friend in my own living room. Two bastards went after Elani over in Israel. She kicked ass. Did I mention that it seems I may be a target as well? Given an informational vacuum, my mind-set is moving toward shoot first, ask later. That being said, what more can you tell me?"

"Ben, I'm sorry as hell. But there's nothing. The details I don't know."

"Well, Stove, let me fill you in. Moore was part of a program to create and train hypnotic couriers and hypnotic assassins."

"I don't know anything about that."

"I'll continue. Both of us know you are lying. You didn't have enough time to practice your story. You just denied information you shared a few minutes ago. The notion is to create people who will learn a message or a mission in one state of mind, and not know the info or their orders in their usual or some other states of mind. If things are set up just right and conditioned very skillfully, the hope is that if these kind of folks are detained, they'll be impervious to interrogation and torture."

Another silence. Two sighs. Stover spoke, "Yeah, I slipped. But you added more. I don't know where you got it. Neither of us is in mid-season form."

"Look, Stove ... and fuck you for holding back when the safety of people I care about is on the line ... This whole project is as secret as the Pope being Catholic. An early researcher spilled the beans in a book on hypnosis a long time back. Everyone pretends he was full of it. But even if I didn't know that, I would have been able to deduce the training from the way this guy has been acting."

"Ben, no one told the Committee about that book. And nobody thought anyone outside that program could figure it out."

"I'll sleep better tonight knowing that!"

Tomasso cut in. "You mean Ben broke in to a secret conditioning protocol that was supposed to be unbreakable?"

Stover's sigh was audible, and followed by a second. "Yeah. I have only one question, Ben. Did you use your training from Israel to break that code? Is Mossad on to this?"

"No to the first. Of course Mossad could figure it out. But with that book out there and Scheflin and Opton's stuff, so could the Uruguayans and Sri Lankans and the Swiss Guards at the Vatican and the Constabulary of Liechtenstein."

"Seriously, Ben. I'm sitting here hoping that you're the genius Tomasso says you are and no Tom, Dick, or Harry could figure it out. Shit-can the modesty. You're scaring me."

"Detecting this stuff is more challenging than the stuff itself. Is it reassuring to know that I drew on my knowledge of hypnosis, psychoanalysis, and psychotherapy research, and that not many people have all those forms of expertise in depth?"

"Well, that's something."

"False reassurance at best. But actually, Stove, there is another factor. Something came up about this case in my department, and all of a sudden some research dork named Will Rivers got hot and bothered to interview him. And when he did see him, he did what I would call some weird shit, and the patient seemed to freak. So although I suspected it from the get-go, I guess maybe the way Will conducted himself threw my misgivings into high gear. By the way, his work is funded by the foundation you declined to name, Glenville-Rodgers.

"What do they do?" asked Tomasso.

"Didn't Stove say they collect senators?" offered Ben.

"I need to talk this through with someone. I'll get back to you."

* * *

Though Stover hung up, Ben and Tomasso stayed on the line.

"Damn, Ben! I don't like this. What do you think he'll get back to you about?"

"All bets are off. Some spook was listening in on us."

"How do you figure that?"

"I may be wrong. But how often does a person sigh twice in succession?"

"What?"

"Seriously. Stover sighed a lot, but sometimes one right after another."

Tomasso found himself sighing involuntarily. Only once. "Oh, shit! I see what you mean."

"I figure some super-spook was listing in, counting on his self-control. He was already on the phone when Stove called you. He said nothing, but I think that every now and then I could hear his reactions.

"When do think Stove'll call?"

"As soon as a real CIA team has me under surveillance and my phones are tapped. I can't wait. And I can't trust him."

SIXTY-FIVE

Ray Hawkes realized he had read the same page of his novel for the third time, and remembered nothing. He tossed the book away in disgust.

Bobby Gray arrived, as always the unshakeable personification of youthful energy and optimism. "Jeff and Ben sent me to give you a hand, Ray. How goes it?"

"So far, so good. I'll be discharged later today. I'm kind of concerned about Eve and Ben. I expected to hear from them."

Bobby looked away from Ray's gaze. "Ben did try to leave you some messages. But Jeff felt you had more than enough on your plate. Don't worry about getting home. I'm your ride."

"But …"

"You just saved Eve's life. The residents decided to pull some shifts helping you out for a while."

"I don't really need …"

"If you pull that 't'warn't nuthin', ma'am' cowboy hero shit we'll put two residents on you full time. They're sending you home on crutches, but that's stupid 'cause you were shot in the shoulder, too."

"You're safe, Bobby. But I'm no cowboy hero. In fact, I'm Apache."

Bobby's big blue eyes widened. "Well, that leaves me completely out of smart-ass remarks. I didn't know."

"Good segue, Bobby. Back to basics. Eve? Ben? Now, Bobby!"

SIXTY-SIX

"So, Rob," Tomasso concluded, "Stover says several former operatives have been linked to this Moore character. He has Americans out front, but there's a United Nations of slime-balls and well-funded professors on his payroll. Inform Ben."

"Got it."

Rob Silverberg was the founder and CEO of SuperGeeks. As a young man, he anticipated that computerization would sweep the world. Rob got so far ahead of the curve and so good at what he did that, in his own words, he became "rich as hell."

Rob, Tomasso, and Ben grew up together. Rob and Tomasso quickly parlayed their brains and skills into impressive fortunes. Both were delighted and less guilty about their success when Elani Enterprises took off, and Elani's success in the fashion industry made Ben a comfortable man.

Ben left Eve Gilchrist at Rob's virtually fortified home, protected by guards and a fantastic security system.

Rob had never lost his boyhood fascination with the old West. When he was teased about it, he shot back, "I got rich as hell so I can be a cowboy any time I want." Rob contemplated the Frederic Remington bronze on his desk, his iconic *Bronco Buster*. Tonight it brought him neither pleasure nor distraction. He began to pace.

"I'm worried. For Ben and for you. Ben has a lot of skills, but ... I don't know. Are you involved with some agency or branch of the military?"

"I'm one of his residents. Just a humble scut-monkey who got caught up in this."

"From your appearance, I thought you might have been one of Elani's girls."

"Elani's girls?"

"The in-house models she hires to show her originals to A-listers in her office."

"I assume that's a compliment. Thanks. I'm not a model. Think of me as Dorothy, just trying to get her bearings in Oz. I'm not sure who is a good witch, and who is a bad witch. Is it OK for me to know what you meant when you said Ben had a lot of skills?"

Rob chuckled. "Probably." He paused.

"Did you know that Ben is a pilot in the Air Force Reserve? Once he served with the IDF."

"No, I didn't. The IDF?"

"Israel Defense Forces."

"So?"

"Ben developed quite a reputation for being effective."

Eve shuddered. "He doesn't seem like that kind of guy."

"Well, turn it around."

"What do you mean?"

"A couple of weeks ago would you have believed that you would take down two trained killers in under sixty seconds, shoot a third in the ass, and keep your Bruno Maglis dry? We forget too quickly. My parents, Ben's parents, Stover's parents—that generation went off to World War II or sat home praying for the boys who did. My dad parachuted into France behind German lines on D-Day and got shot twice taking out a tank. All of these good men took lives, or damn well tried to. When Ben was in Israel, he fought Israel's enemies."

"Someone in the department said he was a killer, that he was put in jail for murder."

"No. Not murder. Just homicide. A man was trying to rape his friend Tomasso's sister. Ben broke it up, and accidentally killed him."

"But these people after us? They're trained killers, aren't they?"

"Ben has some moves. That's all I can say."

They sat in thoughtful silence, pretending to watch the news on Rob's giant TV. Rob assumed that Ben had backtracked to the vicinity of Perth Amboy, New Jersey, knocked on the back door of the Pan-Hispanic Athletic Association, and driven off in a ratty-looking used car with a lot under the hood, a specialty of their old friend Carlos Diaz and his hulking partner Monty Villeneuve.

Some time later they heard a sound that startled them. Someone had knocked at the door of the very room in which they sat.

Ben stuck his head into the room and waved.

"How the hell did you walk past my guards and the best security system money can buy?"

Ben inclined his head and pounded his chest lightly.

"Mea culpa! Mea maxima culpa! Thanks, Rob. We never were here."

"Of course not. Some friend you are! You never drop by, you never call, you never write, you never show up on my surveillance tapes. I assume you've seen Carlos. Here's some info from Tomasso. *Vaya con dios*."

Ben scanned the note, nodded, crumpled it, and tossed it into Rob's wastebasket with a graceful hook shot. He handed Eve a dark baseball cap.

"Time to saddle up, cowgirl!"

Eve waved goodbye to Rob. She and Ben slipped out into the night.

SIXTY-SEVEN

Ben drove north, weaving across interstate and local routes.

"May I ask what we're doing? How on earth do you plan to find him?"

"I don't know. But I have a few ideas about how he'll go about finding us."

Eve chewed her lip, thoughtful and silent. Then she took a moment to fix her lipstick.

"Ben Jordan, you're completely full of shit!"

"Oh?"

"Two can play your game. I've been tracking what you say and how you say it. You go for active solutions. He'll find us because you're trolling for him. You're a fisherman. You're going fishing."

For a few moments Ben seemed to be stifling a cough. Then he burst out laughing. He pulled the bill of Eve's cap down over her eyes and shook her head affectionately, the way he would when a little leaguer came back to the dugout after hitting a home run.

"What have I done? What kind of monster have I created?"

Eve straightened her cap and stuck out her tongue in the dark.

"Payback is a bitch! Suffer!"

She could see Ben shake his head as he laughed. He chuckled for a long, long time.

SIXTY-EIGHT

The Program lost Ben somewhere in New Jersey and missed his transfer to the second car. But its strategists reasoned that as the hour grew late and filling stations closed on minor roads, Ben Jordan might have to stop at a service area on the Connecticut Turnpike.

An operative was relieving himself into a paper coffee cup when he glanced up briefly and nearly soiled himself. Eve Gilchrist was walking from a nondescript sedan into the service plaza. He recorded its license number and waited. Jordan had slipped in unnoticed, but walked out with Eve. The operative reported in and tailed them at a discreet distance. He knew he could have killed one or both, but his orders were to observe and track. The Program hoped the two could be captured and interrogated before being terminated, and preferred that their termination could be accomplished without creating a high-profile event. That meant a private contained setting. Too bad things went wrong at Jordan's house.

SIXTY-NINE

A nameless private road abuts on a major traffic artery on Martha's Vineyard. It appears to be a crude dirt road going nowhere. One hundred feet in, it seems to reach a dead end, but actually angles sharply to the right before sweeping gently back to the left. Arcing back, it plunges into a wooded area, curving gently back and forth, offering drivers a pleasant unfolding display of local flora rather than confronting them with a straight but unsightly earthen gash carved into the countryside. Gradually, hints of less subtle landscaping become evident. Well-selected plantings blend harmoniously with native trees and bushes. Beyond, a lake gradually becomes visible through the trees. Other roads branch off, each wending its way toward the water.

This secluded enclave zealously preserves its obscurity and anonymity. It remains the province of a small number of extremely affluent high-profile families who treasure their privacy. Across the lake from a reconstructed French chateau on the crest of a small man-made rise lies a large single-level home set back from the water. Dense evergreen plantings ensure its near invisibility from the lakeside, the roads, or most of its own grounds twelve months a year. What appears to be a stream feeding into the lake is an artful channel, the entry to a boathouse itself enclosed within a grove of taller evergreens. Naturalistic irregular openings in the foliage around the home allow scenic vistas from its glare-free picture windows, but offer no hint of the structure the landscaping conceals.

In the largest room in this very large house, sunken below ground level, over two dozen men sat around a large table in comfortable task chairs. Fit and neatly dressed, most were in their mid-twenties to early forties. A certain sameness in their clothing suggested some unusual commonality.

Johnson stood as he addressed them. A bandage covered the bridge of his nose. Marty Franks sat subdued, his face badly bruised. Two others sat with swollen jaws. They never opened their mouths.

"We are a small, select group. Some among us volunteered for and received additional specialized training. That training involves a degree of discomfort and risk, but offers the possibility of outstanding rewards.

"Until recently, everything proceeded without incident. We understood some day something might go wrong. We knew that should that day come, we would spare no effort to protect and rehabilitate those who suffered some unanticipated difficulties. No effort or expense will be spared to make things right. We are sworn to leave no man behind."

There were nods of approval all around the table.

"There are folders at your places. Please open them now. The first person pictured is Joe Morgan, known among us as Nicholas Gregorides. We must find him, return him to our training facilities, and if possible, provide for his rehabilitation and return to duty. Hopefully, he's simply confused, and will come back willingly. Whoever locates Gregorides, try to call in Marty Franks, his contact operative. You'll hear from Marty in a moment. If Gregorides resists, take all necessary measures to extract him. Unfortunately, should we fail it will be necessary to eliminate any threat he poses to the Program. Understood?"

Nods all around.

"Before we move on to some other aspects of the mission and our logistics, I want to clarify matters of uniform. I know, I know ..." He waved off their smirks.

"We usually work in small cells. We want to be sure we know who is who. We use indicators like Masonic rings or articles of clothing. A couple of years back we placed a series of orders with L. L. Bean for a particular shirt in many different colors. It's no longer being sold. If anyone else is wearing the same kind of shirt, theirs won't be brand new with the original folds and bright colors.

"Most are blue. Those issued the red print version are most experienced in our methods, like Murdoch, Franks, and Hamner here. Turn to them with questions. Follow their orders without question. The yellow version has been issued to technicians under Junior's direction. Tonight they deploy on diversionary missions.

"We'll walk down the major streets leading to the harbor in Nantucket, solo or in pairs. Upon reaching the harbor, reverse your assigned routes and keep circling and searching.

"Yellow team is go for 0300. Blue and red teams embark 0700 hours. Our equipment is stashed in golf bags. If you need to explain yourselves, you are here with your employer, International Logistic Solutions, for a golf outing.

"We anticipate Nick G. will be wandering around, somewhat confused. We'll move in, sweep the area, extract him, and transport him out in a launch standing off Nantucket Harbor. Worst-case scenario, neutralization with profound regret.

"We hope to avoid the use of deadly force. Only a few senior personnel will go in armed. When you disembark, you will see your transport, the dark blue SUV that carried equipment for our yellow-shirts, and a white van with a Massachusetts license plate. The number is in your folder. The van will bring our 'golf clubs' along.

"Parking has proven a dilemma beyond our logistic capabilities. Once the van is parked, communicate its location. Standard gear."

"A white van?" someone remarked. "There'll be a bunch of them."

"Precisely! Less conspicuous. Anything else? No? OK. Enter, explore, execute, exit."

"And if we can't find him?" asked a man.

"Another team, hopefully unnecessary, will clean up loose ends.

"Now ... Some possible complications. Our host," said Johnson, "informs us that the president received dangerous misinformation from a congressman who is his personal friend. Our people succeeded in preventing any mobilization against us, but the president has asked this man, Representative Elias Stover, to be his eyes on Nantucket. Stover was already nearby, visiting a fisherman from New Bedford he served with in the SEALs."

"SEALs" generated anxious glances and muttering among the men.

"Yeah! Someone like us is in Congress!" Johnson got the laugh he hoped for. Their nervous stirring came to a halt.

"If we encounter Stover, we will convey the president's instructions—for the moment, he is to remain under our protection. If he resists, apologize but insist that you must follow the commander-in-chief's orders. Just tag along with him protectively until you're called off.

"Next are the pictures of Drs Benjamin Jordan and Eve Gilchrist."

Eve's picture evoked appreciative nods and whistles. Ben's did not.

"We hope that they can be captured and interrogated before their probable terminations. We want to know everything they know, and whom they may have told about whatever they've learned, inferred, or guessed. Gregorides began to get impatient about his headaches and went off the reservation. At a student health clinic he was assigned to Dr. Gilchrist. Dr. Jordan became her consultant. He has an interesting background. He could be one of us. His best friend was with Stover in the SEALs. Teams are on the lookout for them.

"Night before last, two of our best isolated Gilchrist at Jordan's house after conning her guards. We don't know what happened, but the bottom line is that Gilchrist killed both just before I arrived. I got her contained and cuffed. Then someone jumped me from behind. We fought. He went down, and I shot him twice, but I was carrying light. We didn't know this other guy was there, or who he is. He has a punch like a mule's kick and runs like a snail. I owe him one.

"Eve Gilchrist is a crack shot and packs a mean punch for a gal. She's Nick's doctor, so he may recognize her and listen to her, despite his training. If we must eliminate her, forget she's pretty. She killed two of our top operatives. Kill her before she sees you coming.

"Jordan is dangerous. Disregard any disparaging remarks in your reports. He's as good as any of us, and battle-hardened. Two of our best tried him and got their asses kicked. Avoid him. Even if you have him outnumbered, do not, I repeat, do not engage him hand to hand. If it comes to it, he should be shot at a distance."

A tall man recruited from SAPO, Sweden's counterintelligence force, spoke up.

"I know of this man. But he must be past his prime by now. Are you sure he deserves such respect?"

"Well, Lars, what would you do if a few years from now someone said something like that about you?"

Lars chuckled.

"Yeah. Point taken. Afterwards, I would send nice flowers."

"Jordan probably cracked aspects of our conditioning modules and could throw a monkey-wrench into Nick Gregorides's training. Keep him away from Nick.

"Memorize your materials. They'll be collected and destroyed before we ship out. Get a good night's sleep. We've lost one of our own. We want to bring him home. Let's have a surgical strike. No collateral damage!

"Anything from you, Franks?"

"Just to back up two things Johnson said. First, call me in when you find him. Second, I went a round with Jordan, Lars. Just shoot him."

"Murdock?"

"I'll be floating and trouble-shooting. Be careful out there. Amateurs are unpredictable."

"Hamner?"

"I'll be walking a perimeter, armed, and ready." He held up a Western-style Colt with pearl handles. Holstering the revolver, he removed a small leather pouch from his pocket. "I took this off the bravest man I ever killed … Just before I killed him. Come back with something to keep from this Ben Jordan. Sooner or later, he has to go."

SEVENTY

Bobby helped Ray into the coach house. After he finished putting away Ray's groceries, he found Ray dragging a duffle bag out to his car, hobbling along with a crutch.

"What are you doing?"

"Ben's out there digging and watching over Eve. Who's got his back? I owe him big, Bobby."

"You're in no shape to drive."

"I'll fly to Boston and then to Nantucket with Cape Air."

Ray made some calls.

"Damn! Booked solid! But I got ferry tickets 'cause they had a cancelation."

"When is the ferry?"

"Tomorrow. 8:30 a.m."

"You got to be kidding!"

"Try me."

* * *

As they pulled out of Ben's driveway, Ray asked Bobby what he'd told his wife.

"I told her before I probably would stay over to make sure you were all right. Look, Ray. We both lost our dads in

Vietnam, and we both were lucky enough to wind up with great stepfathers—both career military guys. As far as we're concerned, this is our fight, too. You damn well better sleep most of the way. In return, I promise to crash and keep out of your hair once we're there."

SEVENTY-ONE

Despite their political differences, Representative Stover and the president enjoyed one another's company. From time to time Stover conducted prayer breakfasts for the president's staff or conclaves of political figures. The president consulted him occasionally, but more often he invited Stover to the White House or Camp David just to join him and a few others to watch a movie or football game.

Stover shared what he'd learned with the president. "This may be a tempest in a teapot, Mr. President. But Jordan is solid and thoughtful. He figured out our most classified stuff just like that. You may hear from folks trying to tell you it's all nonsense. My Committee has seen documentation that supports what he's saying. I'm concerned. By the way, the young woman involved is the daughter of Arthur Gilchrist."

"A friend and strong supporter! Well, Rev, I've already seen quite a parade of visitors beating that nonsense drum loud and long. They say Jordan's own chairman and this hot-shot researcher think he's gone off the deep end."

"That's about as likely as you proposing a round of new taxes on your most generous supporters."

"Point taken. Rev, you've always been straight with me, and you deserve the same in return. Without real evidence, we have a he said/she said, good shrink/bad shrink situation. But who's the good shrink? Who's the bad shrink? My people feel Jordan isn't credible. But I've been briefed above their clearance levels. Your man is on target. That puts me between a rock and a hard place. I can't support him without betraying state secrets and alienating major contributors.

"I hate to ask this of you, Rev. You and Mark are on vacation with an old friend while Liz and your daughters are down at Disney. You're calling from Massachusetts, right?

"How would you feel about catching up with Jordan and being my eyes and ears? I'll give you a number that's good 24/7, except during that conference in Belgium coming up. I'll inform the FBI and CIA that you're acting for me and instruct them to give you whatever you ask for. They'll send liaisons."

"Of course, Mr. President. I'll have to tell Cabral. I can't ..."

"Rev, if I didn't trust your judgment, we wouldn't be having this conversation."

SEVENTY-TWO

The operation went off smoothly. One sniper team identified Ben's car on a rural road, passed, and matched his speed, cruising twenty car lengths ahead.

A few miles later, Ben pulled up behind that team's car at a stop sign. Two shots shredded the passenger-side rear tire.

Masked men stormed out of roadside woods and poured out of the car ahead, weapons trained on Ben and Eve. A man gestured for Ben to roll down his window.

"Joe sent us. Go back where you came from. You'll be in our sights until you hit 476 in PA. Pop your trunk."

One man searched Ben's trunk. He held up Ben's Glock, and nodded to the others. The men from the first car drove off. The rest faded into the woods.

* * *

Eve stood watch as Ben struggled to loosen the lug nuts. Vague sounds came from across the road. Then men were walking toward them. Every man carried a can of beer, and a few bore weapons. A Harley Fat Boy roared up, and aimed its headlight at Eve and Ben. Ben made out nearly a dozen figures. He saw a map of Vietnam on the backs of several vests or jackets.

A very large man with a bushy beard seemed to be their leader.

"Well, I guess those shots messed up your party, too."

"You bet. Not my kind of fireworks," Ben replied.

"You have some problem making friends?"

"Apparently."

Three other men crowded around.

"Glad to see you guys," said Ben.

"Yeah? We could be Hell's Angels."

"You had me worried at first."

A wiry man emerged from the woods where the Program's men had hidden.

"Any of 'em left, Rat?"

"No trace, Spider. Crusty, Cracker, 'n me swept the zone."

Two powerfully built bearded men, one blond, one grizzled, came out of the trees.

Spider turned to Ben. "All recon boys. OK. What the hell is going on here? And who's the Playmate of the Year?"

Eve moved very close to Ben's side. Ben squeezed her shoulder.

"Don't confuse style with substance. These are the good guys."

"We don't hear that too often," said Rat.

"Lot of assholes out there."

"So," Cracker asked, "how did you two wind up getting shot at?"

"They must be communist agents."

"That voice in the dark is Crusty," said Rat.

"We were just driving up to the Cape," Ben tried.

"Consummate bullshit!" Rat snapped. "Try again. You're on a third rate road in the middle of nowhere in the middle of the night. You could have picked half a dozen better routes. Nobody needs nearly ten men to shoot out a tire in the middle of fuckin' nowhere for no fuckin' reason. That's no MO for asshole thrill-killers or crazy kids. This is something weird. Truth time!"

Ben studied Rat. His gut, his training, and his experience shouted, *No way to fool this man!*

"OK. Here it is. There's a guy, former USMC. He's a student at the U in Philly. Came to student health with weird memory problems. Sorry, Eve is not the Playmate of the Year. Natural mistake! She's the psych resident he was assigned to. I'm director of training there. I was called in to consult. We found his notions about what his life had been were inaccurate. We began to pull on some loose threads. It looks like he was manipulated in some spooky research project to transform him into some kind of courier or hit man who wouldn't know what message he carried or the nature of his mission unless someone used the right code to open him up. Dark side of hypnosis.

"Well, fuck us! He wasn't just some messed-up guy fucked over and turned loose. He was still being handled. Somebody got upset, turned him against us, and sent some creepy CIA types for good measure. Sometimes he sees us as his targets, sometimes he knows we're trying to help him. We're trying to stay alive and pull his ass out of this shit. We think we can find what we need to know in Massachusetts. Probably around Bristol County, the Vineyard, or Nantucket."

"Spider, I believe him," Rat spoke up, "There was this guy ... Weird as this shit is, I know ... I can't say how. I just know he's righteous." Rat turned away, sat down, and sipped the beer Crusty handed him. Almost too softly to be heard, he muttered, "It never fuckin' goes away."

Spider sat quietly for a minute, then he nodded to no one in particular.

"Everybody here served. Let's finish our beers, help these folks put on their spare, and take 'em to the state line. Don't know too many folks who'd want to mess with a dozen bikers who look as refined as us."

SEVENTY-THREE

Just before dawn, Ben pulled into the garage beneath his summer home on the western bank of the Childe River in Falmouth. He unloaded a duffle bag and knapsack of his own and two suitcases and a duffle bag for Eve, traveling light, and brought them down to his dock. His old Bayliner lay motionless in the still unruffled morning calm.

Ben boarded silently, the boat brushing gently against a fender. He folded and stowed the tarp over the boat's cockpit, bailed out, and wiped the boat down. He topped off his gas tank. He threw more gear into his knapsack, including a collapsible fishing system with tough resilient line. He tied on a large plug, its array of strong treble hooks protected with corks.

Finally, he checked a forward compartment for an old friend. His Glock had been taken. Earlier that summer, Elani and Ben relocated their weaponry from Childe River before lending their place, but not their boat, to friends whose kids seemed capable of getting into anything. But now he was not completely unarmed.

Eve stumbled down to the dock, stretching and yawning. Looking from the water toward Ben's favorite retreat, and then out toward the bay, she smiled.

"Your place looks wonderful. I'd love to see it when the sun's up. I'd kill for a great cup of coffee. Oops! Bad choice of words?"

"Chop away potentially upsetting words and you're left with grunting like an ape. Coffee in Nantucket."

"Why not take the ferry?"

"They'll be watching for us. We'd be easy to make boarding a ferry. We're traveling low profile."

"Won't we wake up the world motoring out?"

"Maybe not."

Ben wheeled out an ocean-going electric trolling motor and battery on a modified hand truck. It attached to a custom mount at the stern.

"A friend recharged the battery for me last week. We'll sneak out beyond these houses and shade toward the east shore. As we near the bay, no houses on the east shore and just a handful of places on west. We want to be there before the wind comes up."

"There?"

"Nantucket Harbor. Coffee. Sleep on the way."

* * *

Ben shoved off. Once under way, Eve built herself a nest among their duffle bags, and fell asleep in minutes. The electric hummed softly as Ben finessed their way down the Childe. At the river's mouth he switched to gas power. The Bayliner broke gently through the meeting place of tides and currents, where the river insisted upon making its way to the sea, and the sea pushed back, surging toward the shore.

Ben pulled on a sun-bleached fisherman's cap and savored the early morning peace. It seemed to him that some bewildering but inexorable tidal wave of events was racing toward them without his knowing their who, their why, their where, their when, or their how. Gazing to port, he enjoyed a precious few moments of the sunrise. Then he set his course, making for Nantucket Harbor.

SEVENTY-FOUR

Ben and Eve breakfasted and arrived at Coach MacDonald Fletcher's home in time for Ben's meeting with Mack and Coach Buchholz. Jill Fletcher took one look at Eve and bundled her upstairs.

"I hope you like pink," said Jill, settling her into what had been their oldest daughter's room. After a shower, Eve decided to trim down all her nails rather than leave broken and long nails side by side. Despite her morning coffee, she fell deeply asleep in the pinkest room she had ever seen.

Coach Buchholz arrived just after Eve went upstairs.

"Hi, Mike!" said Buchholz. "The family's off to the beach. I guess you're the notorious Dr. Jordan."

"Guilty as charged. Call me Ben."

"How was your trip up, Ben? You've had your adventures."

"Sadly, more of the same."

"Sorry to hear that."

"I want to keep my adventures far from your families. But I need your help.

"The more I know, the better my chance to get Peter Souza back on his feet, and get this craziness under control."

"I checked like you asked," Mack said. "All Pete's brothers and sisters are off-island, scattered to the winds. My son Sean probably knows Pete best. He's a surgery resident at Yale. He caught an emergency case last night … Still in the OR. He'll be here later."

"I can use everything you can remember and everything you can think up or even speculate about Peter Souza."

Coach Mack shared what he knew about Peter, his football career, his friends, and his family. Buchholz had little to say directly, but was helpful in prompting Mack. All three tried to anticipate what Peter might or might not do. Buchholz finally suggested, "Tell him about Peter's best plays. Anything that might have made him really proud and made other people take notice. That might come in useful."

Coach Mack smiled. "It's been a long time. But one really stands out. There was a time when our quarterback, Hawkeye—yeah—don't laugh. Everybody loved *MASH*. Well, I called a quarterback sneak but the defense read it right. Hawkeye was left scrambling around. This big defensive back was just about to tackle him for a loss when Peter comes out of nowhere, throws an incredible block, and Hawkeye scampers in for the score. They gave Hawkeye the game ball, but right while they were taking pictures, he handed it to Peter. Hawkeye told the press Peter deserved it. He said, 'With a block that good, my kid sister could have run it in!'"

SEVENTY-FIVE

Ben was leaving the Fletchers' when their phone rang. Jill called, "Ben, it's for you."

He found himself talking to Ray Hawkes.

"How did you find me?"

"Not that hard. You were going to Nantucket. Joe's case notes say football was really important to him. Given that Nantucket has no pro football team, no college team, and one high school team, and the high school has only one coach, I didn't need rocket science."

"Sorry to get weird on you. Don't I seem to remember you just got shot?"

"Twice, even. I'm supposed to be out of action. I know almost everything about the case, though I've never seen Joe, and vice versa. I'd recognize the bastard that got away. Maybe I can help."

"And if I try to persuade you …?"

"Do you enjoy spitting into the wind?"

"OK, OK! So I am cursed with a great friend … Hey, Ray! Wait a minute! What did you mean, you know the case?"

"It's a long story."

"Talk short."

"Precis: Jeff ordered me to take over the Joe Morgan case. He must think that's his best shot at getting you and Will to stop trying to kill one another. He didn't tell you?"

"No. I wonder if he put you on alert when he was intent on proving I was nuts, and backed off when he saw Joe's story had some basis in fact."

"That makes sense."

"Where are you now?"

"On a boat. Someone let me use their car phone."

Oh, shit! Ben groaned silently. *He really is coming!*

"No way you got home late yesterday, turned around, and drove all night. Who was behind the wheel?"

"Bobby Gray."

"Shit, Ray! He's just a kid. Turn around."

"I don't think you can do that on a Nantucket ferry."

"Make sure Bobby stays out of the line of fire."

"Where do you suppose that might be?"

* * *

Coach Buck came over to Ben.

"Do you want me to do anything?"

"I'd like you to stick close to the Fletchers and my resident. If Peter comes here, send for me. So far, I'm still sorting things out. Some bad guys are after Peter. They want to be sure that they cover their tracks, even if that means getting rid of my resident and me. I want to keep my distance 'cause I'm targeted. I don't want to put others in harm's way. I'll feel better if I know you're near my resident."

"Ben, Jill Mack said that her name is Eve Gilchrist. Is that right?"

"Yeah."

"Her dad some big diplomat?"

"That's the one."

"It's a small world. We'll talk later. You know that I have another thing I have to do. Then I promise you I'll do everything I can. I've got some experience in this kind of thing, from way back, and I'm used to following my gut. I hope it won't screw things up if I follow my own instincts?"

"So this ain't your first rodeo?"

"Not quite."

SEVENTY-SIX

Ben picked up a rental car and drove to where he had docked the Bayliner. He opened the package he'd hidden away, and honed his old friend on a whetstone.

He visited Peter Souza's elderly grandfather at the whaling museum. Philippe Souza said little beyond his direct answers to Ben's questions. But as he grasped what had befallen his grandson, his weathered face slowly took on an expression of unnerving ferocity. *Old or not,* Ben thought, *that is one tough customer! I pity the man who'd cross him.*

Leaving the dock, Ben saw a magnificent custom chopper parked nearby and crossed the street to admire it. A fantastic white stallion galloped across the gas tank. A row of facsimile silver bullets adorned its black saddlebags. He heard a very soft sound behind him and turned quickly, Bowie knife ready.

Even as he turned, a falsetto voice began, "Oh, please don't steal my chopper, Mister Bad Man!" Then, in a gruffer voice, "Geez. You are one fast motherfucker! And you got a new toy."

"Rat? Is that what you look like in daylight?"

"Yeah. Pretty grim, eh? Ain't you gonna ask me why I'm here?"

"No. I see Silver. You're the fuckin' Lone Ranger. You don't like what you heard."

"It really sucks, man."

"Thanks. I knew you were the real deal."

"You got some other Mounties?"

"What do you mean?"

"I can smell pigs. I passed two in a car with a Pennsy plate. A third guy was with them. He looked mobbed up."

"Affirmative. But keep it to yourself."

"Anybody else?"

"Well, funny I called you the Lone Ranger. I have a friend those bastards shot twice and he's coming up anyway. He's an Apache."

"That's a man I'd want on my side. Don't make the cheap joke."

Ben smiled. "That requires a lot of willpower. I'm glad you're here. A bunch of folks are meeting at the police station at eleven. Be there, if only so you won't be misunderstood by the others."

"You mean some might take one look at me and figure my boat ain't moored at the very best yacht club on the island?"

"Something like that. Later."

SEVENTY-SEVEN

Jim Cabot ran the gauntlet between his jeep and the Fletchers' front door. No luck! There was Sarah, Mack's youngest, with a giggling trio of her pre-teen friends. "Hey," Sarah screamed, "It's my brother's hot friend! Doctor Gorgeous!"

Jim bowed to the girls. Sarah offered a mock curtsey in return, and stuck out her tongue.

"Mack? It's Jim."

"Come on in. Sean's not here yet. He had to scrub in on … Something about a few feet of someone's gut not getting enough blood."

"Resection of necrotic portions of the small intestine?" Eve asked.

"Well, hello!"

"Jim, this is Eve Gilchrist. She came up with this Ben Jordan, a shrink who's working on a situation that might involve Sean's old friend Pete Souza. Eve, Jim roomed with my son Sean at Yale and Yale Medical. Then he moved north to Hah-vahd."

Jim shook Eve's hand. "Radiology at MGH. A lowly resident."

"Psychiatry peon at the U in Philadelphia."

Jim lifted her hand. "From your short nails, I figured you to be a surgeon. From your skinned knuckles, I figured you to be a bar-room brawler."

"We bar-room brawlers keep our nails short so we don't gouge our palms too much."

"A recent change in policy?" He had noticed the healing gashes.

"You don't miss much."

They remained holding one another's hand and glances well beyond a little too long. Both Fletchers stifled their smiles.

"My jeep's right out front. Let me show you the island."

"Sure, that would be nice." *Why did I say that?* Eve wondered. *We have a place on the Vineyard. I've been here a million times. I could show HIM the island.*

SEVENTY-EIGHT

"Yo! Ben."

Ben turned and saw Pacella with a taller man. Tall continued.

"The tank saw the Barbie walking with some GQ-type. He jumped out to tail them. We were watching over her back home until those bastards suckered us. Seemed like a good opportunity to take some vacation time."

Ben nodded. He'd met Pacella, but Tomaselli had arrived after he left. These were the men Lucco had promised would stand guard over Eve. All three felt played for fools. They wanted payback.

"Thanks for trying, guys. You were up against CIA rogues and CIA wannabes. For what it's worth, I'm not feelin' too spiffy about my own part in all this. Someone shot out one of my tires last night and I almost got us both killed."

"I don't care how big and bad these guys are supposed to be," Tomaselli growled. "You know the rules—fuck me once, shame on you; fuck me twice, shame on me."

Pacella goaded him, "Oh, Frank! Such language!"

"Fuck you. I'm under cover, disguised as a crude motherfucker."

"I wouldn't count on it. You've already been made by a gentleman of the two wheel persuasion."

"The guy with 'Silver' on his tank?"

"Yeah. Forget his Ivy League appearance. He's with us. Walk around for half an hour or so. Get the lay of the land. Let me see your map. The good guys, including the Lone Ranger, are going to get together there," he indicated. "You'll see a guy with bandages. That's Ray Hawkes. He busted the third guy's nose and got shot for his trouble. Dowling's the chief here. I hear he's good people but he just can't believe all this shit. We've stepped into something pretty nasty."

"Are you saying there may be more of them out there?"

"Yeah, and not to mention who knows which way Pete will break …"

"Whatever this takes," said Pacella. "I have daughters around Eve's age. These bastards—they go down! See you in thirty. Come on, Frank! Let's check out shit we can't afford."

SEVENTY-NINE

Ben returned to the Fletchers' place.

"Sorry, but where's Eve? I just heard she's running around with what a keen observer of the human condition describes as 'a GQ type.'"

Seeing the Fletchers' smiles, Ben chuckled. "You don't seem to be worried. What am I missing?"

Coach Mack smiled.

"Sean's friend Jim Cabot dropped over. When he learned Sean was running late, he offered to show Eve the island. My wife thinks there was instant electricity. He's dropping by our local hospital to help out in radiology. You probably could leave a message for him there."

"Can I talk to your wife?"

"Just coming in with more coffee, Dr. Jordan." Jill was a slim, energetic blonde woman with a mischievous smile. "What do you want to know? Mike says you went to Princeton. No! The single wing won't be coming back. What else?"

"Wow! The perfect woman. Beautiful, makes great coffee, and knows football!" Ben was impressed. *Princeton was one of the last two major colleges to abandon the single wing offense. Most guys didn't know that!*

"My Dad coached at Plymouth. What can I say?"

"You married a treasure, Mack! Jill, if you were Jim Cabot, where would you take Eve Gilchrist?"

"I'd pack a lunch, take a walk in the dunes, read the X-rays on the way back, stop for a cold drink, and then home. But since Jim has a conscience that works overtime, he'll probably call a couple of times to see what the score is with Sean."

"Which dunes?"

"Not around here!" Jill pointed to an old framed map on the wall. She tapped a place with her index finger. "Great Point Light. Jim has a jeep. It's a beautiful place, a wonderful ride, and a great place to walk, talk, whatever ..."

"Now, for extra credit. If you were Maryellen Madeiros, where would you be on a day like today?"

"That's easy. Down Easton to the little beach to the left of the lighthouse. She and Pete would go there to talk or whatever. She takes her children there to play most mornings."

"Her husband?"

"My husband doesn't like me to use the kind of words I'd need to describe him. Pete and Maryellen planned to get married when he got out. But then Pete's parents got a letter that said he died overseas, Maryellen was shattered. She tried to pull herself together, and wound up marrying this guy I'll flatter by calling a loser. The best thing that bastard ever did was to drive into a tree. I feel sorry for the tree."

"Jill!" Coach Mack pretended to be shocked.

"Her ex was the kind of man who liked to hurt people. I don't want to imagine what kind of father he'd be. Between losing Pete and this guy's ... stuff, it's amazing that she's doing as well as she is, and that's not great.

"Do you know the place I'm talking about?"

"Yes. Down Easton."

"Right. Do you want me to come with you?"

"Yes. But no way. There might be danger. Thanks."

EIGHTY

On a small beach at the end of Easton Street a dark-haired woman in her twenties sat on a blanket, watching over a boy and a girl playing in the sand. She was very, very pretty. Her children were completely engrossed in the joys of sand, a blue pail, and two plastic red shovels. As she chatted with her youngsters, she wiped away tears and struggled to keep a smile on her face.

"Maryellen Madeiros?"

"Please go away."

"I apologize. This is no time to intrude. But I need to talk to you, even if you don't say a word to me.

"I'm Benjamin Jordan. I'm a psychiatrist from Philadelphia. I'm here because a patient came to us with a confusing story, and then bolted. I'm worried about him. Normally, psychiatrists can't go running around talking about patients and asking about patients. There are rules against it. But when we learn about situations that may endanger particular people, we have an obligation to warn them. I'm here because you may be in danger."

"You're a little too late. He just got done telling me I'm a whore and threatening to kill me. The bastard went that way." She pointed down the beach.

"I'm sorry. Maryellen—can I call you Maryellen?"

"Anything besides 'fucking cunt' would be a nice change."

"I've heard a tape of him tearing into the young woman trying to treat him. I think he's been brainwashed and convinced that anyone important to him in a positive way is dead or no damn good."

"Can that really happen?"

"It takes some doing, but sometimes, for some people. Especially good hypnotic subjects."

"That's Peter!"

"What do you mean?" *How could she know that?*

"High school graduation week—we were somewhere on the Cape with some of our friends …"

"People like Sean Fletcher, Hawkeye, and Merc?"

"You've done some homework!"

"Coach Mack."

"Pull up a chair."

Ben plopped down on the sand.

"We all went to this hypnosis show. Peter was just sitting there and suddenly his hand is rising and he's walking to the stage and … He was very embarrassed and didn't remember a thing."

"Yeah. Hypnosis is very safe as far as benign interventions go. But even then, there can be problems. Negative effects from stage hypnosis are pretty darn common. That stuff should be banned."

"It was three days before he was right again. He was really weird. For a while you'd just say something and he'd act like it was an order."

"Yeah. It's incredibly important to do adequate dehypnosis, and very few people do it well. Peter must have been really vulnerable. Folks can be taught to protect themselves against that vulnerability, though."

Ben watched the children.

"You've done one hell of a job to have those kids being so happy after all of the crap you've been through."

"They're the only joy I have."

"I don't know how things are going to go. I'll do my best to find him and bring him in safely. But bastards who messed him up are after him too. My Plan B is psychiatric treatment. I think their Plan B is to terminate him to keep their work secret."

"My God! Right this moment I hate his guts. But I love him. Sometimes I wish I didn't."

"Understood. Look. I want to stay in touch with you until this gets resolved. It might be a good idea for you and the kids to lay low for a while. Maybe if you have some family somewhere else in the country. Not on the island."

Maryellen gave Ben a sad smile. "You don't know my family. Peter used to call me 'the best of a bad lot.'"

"Abusive?"

"I might answer that after I knew you for a decade or two and got drunk as hell."

"I'm sorry."

"This morning was just horrible." The tears came. "I think my dreams finally just rolled over and died." Maryellen began to shake.

Ben put an arm around her shoulder as she sobbed. The girl asked, "Are you OK, Mommy?"

Ben said, "Mommy is thinking about something sad. Let's let her cry for a minute and I think she'll be OK." Maryellen nodded, and her daughter toddled off.

"It's all just too much! I can't give up one more inch, one more minute of my goddamn lousy life to crazy dreams! But they're all I have left." She sighed. "How the hell would you know what I mean? You don't become some big-shot doctor by starting out as trash, getting squashed, and then being called a fucking whore by the man you wanted to be with forever!"

"Well, I've really worked with a lot of people …"

"Whatever!"

"What a ladylike way of telling me I'm full of shit!"

Maryellen laughed. "Five minutes ago, I never thought I'd laugh again. Are you supposed to be good at what you do?"

"I guess."

"Any words of wisdom?"

"As a matter of fact, yes. Right from Sigmund Freud. He said in smaller matters, let reason and logic guide your actions. But for important things, follow your heart."

"He just said that so fools like me would follow their dreams into heartbreak, get depressed, and have to come to him forever."

"Who knows? I'll float that one by at the next American Psychoanalytic meeting."

"Love can be an awful thing. But then, you probably know that from some book you read. When it really hits, it's hard to make it go away."

"I can't disagree. Once upon a time I walked in on someone trying to rape my best friend's sister. I was trying to punch him in the face, but I slipped on something—hit him too low and fell on my face. I was comforting her and didn't even realize the guy was hurt bad until a few minutes later. He wasn't even breathing. My punch broke his larynx. I wound up in jail.

"Anyway, by the time that got sorted out, the school year was shot. I went over to Israel and spent some time on a kibbutz. One day I was taking a bus somewhere through the desert. I looked out of the window and saw this girl in an army uniform. I bought two bottles of water from someone and got off the bus."

"You've got to be kidding!"

Ben chuckled. "I walked over to her and tried to strike up a conversation. I proposed to her that very day. She thought I was nuts. And after seven years, emigrating to Israel, making an international fool of myself, and chalking up too many rejections to count, she suffered a severe lapse of judgment and married me.

"So, there are those of us crazy people who just don't know how to quit. I think I understand. I hope things work out the way you want."

"How could you keep on going? I mean, I feel like a complete loser. Maybe I'm just too stupid to give up on Peter?"

"I know that feeling pretty well."

"I guess I'll hang on a little longer. It's hard."

"Another day, another ordeal. Meanwhile don't forget your other dreams."

"Another day, another ordeal? Yeah, true. Can you believe that I was just a stupid little girl who wanted to marry Peter and teach kindergarten?"

"No. I can believe that you were a smart little girl who wanted to marry Peter and teach kindergarten. You underestimate yourself."

"No one ever told me that before."

"Shame on them. What do they know? I've got a meeting with the chief of police. I'll keep in touch." Ben waved as he left. He was ten yards down the beach when Maryellen called after him.

"Hey, Dr. Jordan! Thanks."

EIGHTY-ONE

Chief of Police Steven Dowling scrutinized the men assembled before him, as unwelcome and ill-matched a crew as he'd ever confronted. Several seemed to be sizing up one another with similar suspicions and misgivings. Only this Ben Jordan character seemed completely relaxed. Ben told Bobby to take a hike.

"Go see the whaling museum."

"Better still," said Dowling, "go down to the docks and take a whale-watching cruise."

Bobby's face lit up like a Christmas tree. "Whales? Really?"

"Try the *Queen of Lisbon*."

Watching Bobby leave with a near-beatific look on his face, Ben couldn't help but smile. *At least that's one out of the line of fire!*

"Was I ever that young?" Dowling mused. He turned back to the men and gave a long, deep sigh.

"Instead of doing what the taxpayers of Nantucket pay me to do, I'm sitting here with you. I'm not convinced that this is anything more than a—nonsense. And some of you look like you're on the wrong side of the bars.

"You've got ten minutes to make this make sense to me, or you walk out of here as the weirdest bunch of kooks to hit this island. Who's talking?"

Ben raised a hand.

"Chief, you're right. We're quite a collection. There's a young doctor from back in Philly whose office and home were trashed. She was being tortured until I broke it up. Two times I put her in places I thought were safe, but people representing themselves as feds nearly kidnapped her. At my own home they presented legit-looking credentials to two off-duty cops watching over her, and tried to snatch her. Those cops, Pacella and Tomaselli, are here. The big guy there is Lucco Brazzo, a good friend. The fellow over there with the bandages is my friend, colleague, and neighbor, Dr. Raymond Hawkes. Ray heard shots from my place, came running, and got shot twice for his trouble. He saved her. While she and I were driving here someone shot out one of our tires. The gentleman whose presence probably puzzles you the most? He and his friends helped us out and got us back on the road. He's a Good Samaritan, pure and simple."

Ben summarized the background information.

"This Johnson fellow continued developing these specialized operatives, now for hire for big bucks. Our man was in college, probably being established as a sleeper. He went to student health for bad headaches. I got consulted by the young woman assigned to treat him. Johnson and his people have been trying to recover this man and cover their tracks. The young doctor and I are inconvenient loose ends.

"We came to Nantucket because I've identified the fellow in trouble as Peter Souza, an islander reported dead overseas. He actually went or was taken off the grid under the name of Joe Morgan. He doesn't know who he really is. I thought he was likely to come back here. He was engaged to an island girl named Maryellen Madeiros.

"We want to get to him first both to protect him and to treat him. We want to bring this thing to an end because until we do, both he and the young doctor are at risk."

"What about you? And, what about proof?"

"I think what makes them safe will make me safe. Proof? A member of the House committee that oversees our intelligence forces gave me most of this info, some 'Project Nick.' I knew something was wrong, but I didn't know about the cloak and dagger stuff till I reported it up the line. I didn't make up this nightmare, I just happen to be living in it."

Dowling nodded.

"Sounds like complete bullshit to me!"

"I agree."

Ben stood up, handed Dowling a piece of paper, and stepped back, positioning himself along a wall.

"Those are phone numbers for the chief of security at the U, Detective Bleier of the Philly PD who caught the case at the U, the detectives in Lower Merion, and the duty officer at NIS Northeast in Newport, who'll confirm the men who came to my house posing as NIS were frauds. If you think the feds gave me a number, you've gotta be kidding. Feel free to call any and all.

"I have no problem with your thinking I'm crazy. I'm thick-skinned. I would have problems with your not checking out my credibility while armed goons are hunting down Peter Souza and my student doctor on your turf. No cop wants this stuff in his own backyard."

Dowling nodded. He called Newport and didn't like what he heard. He tried to call Lower Merion, but it didn't go through. He shrugged.

"OK. So you're not the weirdest bunch of nut cases ever to hit the islands. But you may be the least welcome. Introduce yourselves."

After intros all around, there was a knock at the door.

"Hi! Chief Dowling?" A young, clean-cut man asked. "Sorry to barge in. I just tried to call, but your phone line seems to be down."

Dowling picked up his receiver. It was dead.

"Hmm. So it is. It'll be restored soon. Sorry. What can I do for you?"

"Herbert Johnson. I was asked to deliver a message on behalf of government agencies."

From the wall, Rat murmured, "Oh Gawd! Spare me!"

"I feel so much better," Pacella was pissed.

"Cool down, Tony. He'll tell us what he wants to, when he's ready," said Dowling. "The message?"

"Someone is en route from Washington to look into the situation here and report back. I was asked to bring you that information."

"Someone?"

"I'm not authorized to be specific."

"Well," Dowling chuckled, "we'll eagerly await the arrival of someone."

Prentice James, a tall African-American volunteer policeman with a perpetually thoughtful expression, ushered in two men.

Representative Elias Stover waved a somber hello and took a seat. The other man resembled Herbert Johnson save for the color of his hair and shirt. His uncreased and aggressively neat casual clothing screamed L. L. Bean-clad upwardly mobile junior fed.

Ben realized that the others didn't recognize Stover.

"Chief, we've just been joined by the gentleman to whom I alluded. Meet Reverend Elias Stover, member of the House of Representatives from Detroit, Michigan, formerly a Navy SEAL."

Dowling welcomed Stover, who stood and looked around the room. The two young feds sat with perfect posture. Ray shifted uncomfortably in his folding wheelchair. Tomaselli,

Pacella, and Lucco Brazzo leaned forward in their chairs. Rat slouched against a wall. Prentice James began to write a note. Ben Jordan sat down alongside James. His arms folded across his chest, he stared hard at Stover.

Stover could only hope that Ben understood his situation. Matters of national security and his president's orders trumped Ben's personal concerns. In military situations, Stover knew he or Ben would obey without question orders that placed their lives in danger. He also knew that if Ben felt the safety of people he cared about was threatened, Ben would regard Stover, the government, and the known universe as enemies if they opposed his efforts. Stover resigned himself to enduring Ben's outrage.

"I wish I had been able to reach you before, Ben, but I couldn't make that happen."

When Ben said nothing, Stover turned to address the men.

"May I, chief?" Stover asked. "I'm here at the request of the president of the United States. I wish that I could tell you I know what's going on. I got tapped because I was already in the vicinity.

"Ben, I passed your input up the line. It wasn't taken seriously in all quarters. Several senators and reps ridiculed your observations. They backed Glenville-Rodgers and assured the president that whatever was going on is nothing of concern. They quoted a prominent behavioral scientist who challenged your concerns and questioned your sanity.

"But other sources confirm your credibility. Among politicians, doubt won by a landslide. Among intelligence analysts it was a Mexican standoff. Half agreed with you.

"These two gentlemen are my liaisons to major agencies concerned with our national security."

He gestured to the second of the two younger men.

"We are going to hear from the gentleman whom you've met, and from Mr. Johnson here …"

Tomaselli, Brazzo, Pacella, Rat, Ray, and Ben groaned as one.

Stover looked puzzled.

"Sorry, Stove," explained Ben. "The first guy already claimed Johnson. One Johnson per misinformation session, please. We've had more than enough CIA Johnsons to last a lifetime. Especially the one with Czisniewski and Minetti."

"Will Jones do?" the first fed ventured. Stover smiled, and Prentice James, his expression blank, passed his note to Dowling.

"We'll call you Nicolai Rimsky-Korsakov," Lucco suggested. Rat seconded the motion.

"That will enhance your empathy with the Nick experience," Ray insisted.

Nicolai applauded his tormentors, winning some points. Dowling shrugged.

"OK! OK, guys! Let's give it a rest. Fill them in, Nicolai."

"We're all ears, Nick!" said Tomaselli.

Nicolai spent five minutes summarizing what everyone already knew, and continued.

"Unsubstantiated reports suggest that said Joe Morgan may have broken away from a control program, code name 'Nick.' He may have made his way to this area, and that this group may have mobilized significant resources to contain and recover him. No group of any size has arrived by either scheduled airlines or charter flights, or ferries. That notwithstanding, if a few men were sent using several different transports, a good-sized team could be assembled.

"The only fairly inconspicuous way to bring a good-sized group to Nantucket this time of year would be a private boat or boats. The harbormaster here connected us to a boat dealership down the way that has a few slips they rent to transients, and others they'll rent if they clear inventory faster than anticipated. The owner reports that two good-sized high-speed motor craft came in earlier today without advance reservations, one shortly after the other. This marina generally handles high-end sailboats. Usually it doesn't get that kind of traffic. They had two slips big enough, but one was reserved for a Morgan Out Islander. Their techs are replacing its radio later this morning. The second one got a mooring. It had a Zodiac in tow. A lot of men came in on them, with a lot of golf bags. He said they all were young, fit, polite, and neatly dressed. Somebody with a white van and another with a dark SUV met the boats. It could be anything from a company, reunion, or convention golf outing up to an infiltration of hostiles dressed—well, like I am."

"Any big groups booked at any hotels or golf courses on the island?" asked Ray.

"Negative. There is one additional piece of information of unknown significance. Yesterday, Mossad informed us that earlier this week two American males posing as CIA operatives approached three Israeli women on the private property of a prominent industrialist with dual US-Israeli citizenship. They tried to coerce a certain Elani Weisenthal to go with them. Whatever went down, they wound up sun-poisoned and in the custody of Mossad. They said they were working for a clandestine unit of the CIA that does not exist …"

The room filled with derisive laughter.

"Really, guys … Really! We don't know what to make of this."

"Give the little kid a break," said Dowling.

"Chief, no way he gets a break!" said Ben. "Elani Weisenthal is my wife. This whole thing isn't happening in never-never land."

"I'm not in a position to share any more. You don't have clearance."

"Not good enough!"

Stover broke in, "Ben, he has his orders."

"Like the second guy on the phone when you called?"

"Shit! How did … Never mind. How did … Never mind!"

"Stover, tell me how your spook club's report, while managing to be so informed about my alleged shortcomings and proudly enumerating the heroic patriots who defend

Glenville-Rodgers, somehow managed to make no mention of police reports regarding the curious happenings in Philly and Lower Merion? You know, where Dr. Gilchrist had her home and office trashed, and where meaningless moments transpired, like when she was being tortured till I broke it up. That's also where she fought off one attempt to kidnap her with an assist from Lucco here, and had to kill two of the three guys trying to kidnap her from my home, which is now a crime scene, to stop another. That's where Ray here went after the third, busted the asshole's nose, got shot twice for his trouble, and acquired that wheelchair. Do these things stir further thoughts?"

"That information is restricted!"

"Restricted! It's all a matter of public record. Check your newspapers. Four people were shot and two died in my house!" Ben's voice was too calm. He rose slowly.

"Ben," Stover tried, "he's following his orders."

"We really need to know what's going on here." Ben's voice grew even milder as he approached Nicolai.

"Oh, shit!" Lucco muttered, "Oh, shit!"

"You're talking about my family and friends. Do you have a wife and kids?"

"No."

Rat could see the next move. *Here it comes!*

Ben's Bowie knife was at Nicolai's crotch.

"Listen, baby spook. This is not your fault, but if you ever want to have a wife and kids, start talking. If you don't there's no one in this room who can stop me from feeding your nuts to the seagulls."

"You can't intimidate me!"

Stover broke in. "I'll be responsible. Tell the man."

"With all due respect, sir …"

"Our commander-in-chief instructed me to call it like I see it. Tell these men. Never underestimate Jordan. Never push him to the wall. I've seen him in action."

"I can take care of myself, sir."

"Please, son. You're one centimeter from a circumcision and two from a voice change. I need you in one piece. So—no, you can't. Not with him."

"On your authority, congressman. The men in Israel told Mossad that they were part of a CIA unit so covert its existence would not acknowledged."

Rat hummed the theme from *Mission Impossible*.

"They said that they were working under the cover of a contractor anonymous to them."

"Bullshit! Who cut their checks?"

"International Logistic Solutions."

"Which led where?"

"I don't know."

Ben stood up again.

"He doesn't know, Ben," said Stover.

"Bullshit! No federal agency, even on its worst day, stops short like that unless it's called off."

"OK, OK. The investigation is incomplete. So far we've found a series of shell corporations chartered in Delaware, operating under legally obtained fictitious names with legitimate bank account and holdings. But since each has a parent company registered in the Caymans, we don't think we're anywhere near the bottom ..."

"What else?"

"That's it."

"Bullshit again! How can someone organize a bunch of reasonably skilled CIA act-alikes, and put them in the field while this remains an unsolved mystery to every alphabet soup federal agency known to man?"

"We don't know."

"No ideas?"

"No."

"Look, are you for real?" Again, Ben was too mild. "I could assemble a crew of people like that without breaking a sweat.

Or I could rent them from some firm that calls itself a private security contractor but can function as a private army."

"That's enough from you, Jordan!"

"But not enough from you, baby spook. What's going on right now all over the country? Anyone here interested in sports?"

Ray burst out, "Oh, shit!"

Ray is quick, Ben thought. *But that quick? Impressive!*

"Tell them, Ray."

"All over the country, NFL training camps are getting started."

"What the hell does that have to do with anything?" asked Nicolai. "Oh, no! I'm an idiot. Training camps ... Or like the waiting list at a good college. Yeah. If I hadn't made the cut, I would have jumped at the chance to join some special off the books secret unit. I get it."

"So, I assume," Ben said, "that what you're not telling me is that perhaps one or both of the men who went after my wife in Israel may have come in off your waiting list, your taxi squad, your whatever ..."

"I cop to being a complete jerk. Yeah! One washed out late in training when he busted up a knee. He had darn good potential. And over here, Czisniewski was ours, but he liked to hurt people too much. Minetti is a bogus name, but his picture matches a special ops guy we thought was dead. He probably went off the grid."

"OK," said Ben. "Get married, make more Nicolais. But now you can understand why these bozos seem to have an unlimited supply of pretty darn good people. Some may really believe they're the good guys. It's a good bet some pretty badass types playing super-soldier are leading a mix of assholes and misguided wannabes.

"A few bribes to personnel/human resources types in key positions in various nations and you could recruit a United Nations of high quality operatives, absolutely loyal and determined to prove themselves to those who've shown confidence in them. I'd say that's nothing short of fucking brilliant. Continue, Nick."

"Nothing more here. Chief Dowling, what would you like to add?"

"We're a community of 10–11,000 islanders. That jumps to 40–50,000 all summer. Our standing police force is small. We bring on part-timers and volunteers in season. We're not equipped to deal with the kind of people you're talking about.

"Earlier today fires were breaking out all over the island. Every last one is so near to a major road and so smoky that my people are still in the field, handling the traffic and chaos. Every piece of fire equipment is out. The airport was shut down because fires were set all along the runway. I have volunteers at the airport and ferry slips keeping an eye on things. But volunteers are trained to handle routine and minor stuff. Not many troops left to rely on. Just me and Preston here at headquarters, and he's a volunteer.

"Another thing. Last night the power and phones went out for about half an hour. The desk officer had to leave the station to call for help. When he got back, the power was back on. He noticed a burning smell. Probably a power surge. Our computer was fried, and the electronics for our weapons locker went nuts. It won't open. We have a call in to our locksmith.

"That leaves us with whatever off-duty guys we can roust with their service weapons, riot guns in the trunks of cruisers scattered all over creation, and whatever you brought with you. Fishermen who go for the big stuff carry guns to put down sharks they can't handle on board, but they'll already be hours off shore."

"Ben," Stover began, "that guy Buchholz who came over to talk to you …"

"Well, he actually was going to be on the island for something personal, but he said he could take some time out to help me."

"Ben, let me finish. The guy has a history. Thirty years in the Marines and he wasn't a quartermaster."

"Your call."

"When you meet him, fill him in."

"To me, this all means that Fletcher, Coach Mack, and his family might be in the line of fire."

Stover was silent. "He has to be told."

Nicolai sighed, shrugged, and nodded.

"What are we overlooking?"

"No one knows what Joe, Nick, or Peter will turn up and what he'll do. Will he make a beeline for home? Will he respond to some cue and fall into line with Johnson/Moore or whatever and come after any of us on cue, or even go after his own family? He's been told they're dead. Those bastards may have tried to convince him his own folks are enemy agents, disguised as the family he loves. Same for the girlfriend. I met her. She's a widow with two kids."

"Eve Gilchrist's whereabouts are unknown. She slept in. Coach Mack told me that his son's friend, Dr. Jim Cabot, whom Lucco described as 'some GQ guy,' is showing Eve around … I know.

"I was stupid enough to let her sleep and figured … But he walks in, they walk out. Fletcher vouches for him."

"Are we missing the big picture here?" asked Brazzo, "What about these other bozos? What's the plan?"

Dowling tried the telephone again. The line was dead.

"I don't know what's going on," said Dowling. "But for the immediate future, we're cut off. We can't count on reinforcements or supplies."

"CB, ham operators, flight controllers, car phones, marine radios?"

"CB is iffy, the only hams I know are off-island right now, airport's evacuated … Only a handful of car phones I know of. Best shot is to go to the Coast Guard station, get to a boat, or send a boat out …

"But until we reconnect with the outside world, we're looking at a situation I don't like. Twenty-plus operatives with weapons we can't match and strong logistic support are combing Nantucket ... This one is a bit over my head."

Stover nodded.

"OK, but we have two trained operatives here ..."

"Well," Nicolai began ...

Dowling broke in. "With all due respect, you look like a rookie to me. You ever run something like this?"

"I've been trained ..."

"So the answer is 'no,'" said Dowling. "Son, Prentice recognizes you. That's why he wrote that note. He works part time at the hotel where you've been staying. You came for your frat brother's wedding and you're staying on a few days with some old friends. Noah, the bartender, says you drink gin and tonics with the house gin. You've acquired a parking ticket and bar tabs under a different name. Your people probably mobilized you because you're already here. No disrespect intended. Tapping you for first aid makes sense. Not sending a more senior person on the next plane or boat means they're not taking things seriously. This is happening on my island, on my watch. That's not good enough."

Stover agreed. "I have confidence in you as an operative, son. But if this is your first rodeo, we can't lay it on you."

He looked to the second young man.

"You hiding years of experience under that unlined boyish face?"

"No, sir!"

Stover looked around.

"Unless I miss my guess, there's only one man in this room who has experience with armed infiltrators among civilian populations."

EIGHTY-TWO

Junior's yellow-shirts began before dawn. As the day went on, dozens of mayday calls from the boats they sabotaged would overwhelm Coast Guard operations.

He reported Congressman Stover's arrival aboard Cabral's *Os Lusiadas*. Johnson instructed him to put Cabral's boat out of commission. Junior motored out of the harbor, came about, and approached his target from seaward, shielded from the sight of those on shore by the angle of his course and the size of *Os Lusiadas*.

EIGHTY-THREE

Ambassador Gilchrist was sitting quietly with a cup of tea when Bill Buchholz walked into the breakfast room of his hotel.

"Thanks for coming, Buck. I can't tell you how much it means to me."

"No problem, Mr. Ambassador. We're in and out of the island all summer. My wife's college roommate has a rambling old house with more than enough room, and the families get along great."

"Well, Buck. You know I can talk all day without getting down to a subject, so I'll force myself to come to the point."

"Yes, sir!"

"Buck, I've taken a long time to get around to straightening out certain aspects of my life. Over the last year I've come to accept that I'm an alcoholic. So is my wife. I guess we've been each other's enablers as well. There are so many of us in the diplomatic corps that we can carry on with our merry dances, sometimes for our whole careers, sometimes for the rest of our lives."

Buck listened.

"So, one day I saw through myself. Not for the first time. This time it stuck. I'm still not sure why, but I called AA. I did my ninety meetings in ninety days. My wife came with me. Thank God, we're as well matched to support one another in sobriety as we were drinking. Our marriage has never been better.

"I won't deny that some days I think the whole twelve step thing is bullshit, but the more I work it, the better things get. Anyway, Buck, I've been working the steps. And now I'm looking at that ninth step, making amends. And I'm thinking that of all the people I owe apologies to, you're at the top of the list. I treated you very badly on many occasions. Like when you taught Cricket to shoot."

"But Mr. Ambassador! You apologized as soon as you were reminded of what you said. You apologized right in front of the staff."

"Yes, Buck, I do know I did. But Buck—I don't remember doing it. I don't remember a damn thing! I had a blackout. No—it's no good to me in my recovery if I don't know in my heart what I did and didn't do. I know that I did that because I was told. But I really don't know that I did that—not from my own experience. For me, for now, I have to know and to hold in my own memory that I did the right thing.

"So, I apologize, Buck. I'm not asking for your forgiveness. I just have to tell you that I know I did wrong, and you didn't deserve it. You're a fine man, Buck. As fine as any I've ever known. You're still my kids' number one hero. And I think the Cricket got a lot of her best qualities from the time she spent with you."

"They remember me? I'm—I'm very grateful. They're all good kids, sir, but I always had a special spot in my heart for the Cricket."

"She still talks about you. She's halfway through a psych residency at the U in Philadelphia."

"This is very mind-blowing, sir. Like I told you, I was already coming to Nantucket on other business, not just vacation. That other business involves helping a psychiatrist trying to treat a guy from around here, some lost soul who stumbled into my office a while back, expecting to find his old coach there. I helped this psychiatrist find the coach the patient was looking for. Turns out he was right here in Nantucket. The doc drove up with a young woman resident who was still asleep when I met with him. Ambassador, that young woman's name is Eve Gilchrist. She's probably the Cricket."

"Oh, my God! I'll have to tell …"

"Mr. Ambassador, some pretty nasty people are after her and this other guy."

"Well. That's really something. Are you sure?"

"Affirmative. If these people know you two are here, they may be tempted to move against you to pressure Eve to give them whatever they want. Jordan asked me to watch over her and the coach's family. He doesn't know the connection."

EIGHTY-FOUR

Ben worked to prevent his face and body from betraying his despair. His hopes that federal agencies would respond to the situation with appropriate manpower and resources were dead. Glenville-Rodgers had convinced some heavy hitting contribution-oriented legislators to intervene. Money, more eloquent than Demosthenes or Cicero, more alluring than Sophia Loren or Marilyn Monroe, once again had demonstrated its unique persuasive power.

Horrible flashbacks swiftly returned him to his personal hell. Electric shock waves seemed to pass through his head, his hands, and his genitals. It was all he could do not to scream and convulse.

Long ago, in Israel, Ben led an operation that relied on disastrously inaccurate intelligence. His squad walked into a deadly ambush. The survivors were handed over to interrogators who went about their business with a vengeance. Will had tried to use this episode to discredit Ben.

Wrenching away from his past, Ben nodded. Stover knew this was no SEAL-type op. The young feds were clueless. While Nicolai had been embarrassing himself, the second had hardly said a word. Was he circumspect or someone to be concerned about? Ben could not afford the luxury of wondering. He put that nagging concern aside.

"I hate to ask this of you, Ben," said Stover. "But I trust you. You've been ahead of the curve and right on target about every single godforsaken thing. We need you."

EIGHTY-FIVE

Ambassador Gilchrist and Buck prepared to depart. Buck would watch over Eve "Cricket" Gilchrist. The ambassador would lay low.

"But before I forget," the ambassador said, "remember when I used to go on about how I wanted to bag the big five and be the great white hunter? And I was determined to own one of those Purdey 'dangerous game' rifles?"

"Sure. You talked a lot about the African big five. And those rifles! Especially when the emir paid a visit."

"Yes. Well, the emir is, was a man of unlimited wealth. One day he came over for a friendly dinner—nothing political. After dessert, he had his man bring in two gun cases. 'Pick either one,' he said. So, I picked one. Then, he said, 'Let's open them.' We did. In front of me lay a magnificent Purdey .470 Nitro Express. We were about the same size. He bought an identical pair. He apologized if the engraving was not quite to my taste."

"The engraving, sir?"

"Well, Buck, a Purdey epitomizes aesthetics and function. Its engraved areas become a canvas in metal. Europeans and Americans usually choose among a variety of hunting scenarios. Being a devout Muslim, the emir felt obligated to avoid representational art. Most Islamic hunters select a pattern called 'large scroll with extra finish.' I promised to show you that gun if I ever got hold of one."

"Sir, that was fifteen years ago. And you said the emir was …"

"That's a long story for another time. But I did make a promise, Buck. I hope I can take you down to the boat and show you the damn thing."

"I'd like to see it, Mr. Ambassador. You came by boat?"

"On the old *Cricket's Caper*."

"How the hell did we keep up with her?"

"We didn't, Buck, but we tried."

"I'm remembering the frogs, sir."

"Spare me that one, Buck." He pulled out his wallet.

"You didn't see her. This is a picture of the monster of yesterday as she appears today, there with her mother."

"My God, Ambassador! Betty hasn't changed, and the Cricket's become a real beauty!" Buck started to reach for his own wallet, and stopped.

"Company," he said.

A clean-cut man in his late twenties wearing a red shirt approached them.

"Ambassador Gilchrist?"

Buck broke in, "Who's asking, son?"

"I've been told not to identify myself unless it is absolutely necessary."

Buck laughed, "We have company with a capital C."

"So, young man," Ambassador Gilchrist began, in his most congenial tone, "What does the Central Intelligence Agency want with an old diplomat on vacation?"

"Perhaps this should be a private conversation, sir."

"Son, Sargent Buchholz has guarded more V.I.P.s and state secrets than you'll ever know. Continue, Mr. uh …"

"Johnson, sir."

"Of course. Don't chuckle, Buck! There actually are people named Johnson. Go on."

"We're trying to determine the whereabouts of your daughter, Dr. Eve Gilchrist."

"What? Frogs in the drinking water again?"

"No, sir. A person who is a threat to national security became a patient of hers. She and some Dr. Jordan went out looking for him. But this guy is a loose cannon, and some bad folks want to catch up to him as much as we do. This Jordan fellow put your daughter in the middle of a dangerous situation."

"So, why are you in Nantucket instead of in Philadelphia?"

"Because we have reason to believe that your daughter is here on Nantucket with that Jordan, trying to find this man."

"That's news to me! I've been sailing offshore. I just stopped here to have a new radio installed."

"I hate to say this, sir, but my superiors were concerned about the coincidence of her arrival here and your own. I'll reassure them."

"You've just told the ambassador that your superiors suspect him of involvement in that something that sounds … like an accusation of treason," said Buck.

"Off the record, I'm ashamed to be here on a mission that I personally consider mindless and offensive. I can extend my personal apologies, but I have to respect my chain of command."

"No offense taken, son. Where can I reach you?"

"I'll catch up with you sometime today."

After the man had left, the ambassador turned to Buck. "I don't like this, Buck."

"I don't much like coincidences, sir. Eve must be that resident I just missed running into. Ben Jordan was consulting on that case. His own departmental chairman put him on the case because he knows a lot about the way the cloak and dagger folks try to manipulate minds, did an about-face, and now he's throwing him under the bus. I read him as solid. What concerns me here is what our last visitor is up to. He seems sincere, but I wouldn't want him on my six."

"Buck, fill me in. Don't spare the details. I'm taking notes. This Jordan? Would you trust him to cover your six?"

"No question. While I want to move on, I have two concerns. First, I'm afraid of being followed and leading them to Cricket. Second, I'm concerned about your safety and security. I think I'd best have another cup of tea."

Ambassador Gilchrist waved to a waitress.

"Restaurant is closed until lunch, sir, but Noah at the bar will be glad to keep things flowing. Just walk to the next room over. I'll clear."

EIGHTY-SIX

Ben regrounded himself.

"You know me, Stove. My track record was less than stellar."

"Your record was stellar. One mission went terribly wrong."

Nicolai broke in. "OK, I've got to know who this guy is."

Finally, the second man spoke. "Yeah. I need to know what to report."

"What's your name?" Rat asked.

"Uh …"

"Don't waste time with the name game," said Lucco, "Just call him Borodin."

"Why?"

"Consider it fate," said Lucco.

Ben and Dowling chuckled with Lucco. Another Russian composer! Borodin's music was the score of *Kismet*, a great Broadway musical.

"Kismet means fate." Dowling smiled, "My wife and I loved that show."

"Colonel Benjamin Jordan, 150th Air Lift Wing, New Jersey Air National Guard."

"Air Force? Oh, shit!"

"Formerly I served in the Israel Defense Forces—counterterrorism."

"Sorry, sir! That works for me."

Dowling sighed. "I'm OK with that. My church group went to Israel a few years back. Their security folks crawled up everyone's ass—more than once. I'm counting on you to do the same."

"Understood," Ben said. "I'll try to be difficult.

"We face several problems. Thus far, our only basis for identifying bad guys is superficially polite behavior and clean-cut appearance observed at a distance. Using search criteria like that, we'd nab Nicolai and Borodin, a bunch of Canadians, a handful of Midwesterners, and maybe a stray Brit.

"We don't know who our enemies are, what assets they possess, or what they actually plan to do. We have limited strength, and even more limited armaments. We have to avoid mission creep.

"We can't just go off like vigilantes. Chief, please deputize everyone. Provide us with badges, Miranda cards, and a baton and cuffs if you can. Tangible indicators of legitimate authority may be our best way to exert influence. We have no meaningful weaponry to distribute.

"For all we know, lots of the people we'll face really believe that they're the good guys. Containment is the key. Isolate, overwhelm, and take more and more of them out of action. No standard confrontations. No firefights.

"Stove! Where's Cabral?"

"He has no clearance for this stuff. He went home."

"Stove, whenever you deal with security clearances, your brains turn to shit. Cabral is a SEAL and exceptionally smart. But, even figuring in his defective judgment in being your friend, I bet he stuck around to cover your ass."

"You ruined my surprise." Six foot six of Annibal Cabral walked in. "Yeah. I sent the boys home with the boat."

There was a burst of laughter from behind him. Cabral turned.

"I told you to go home. Ahh!" He raised his hands to the heavens. "Kids!"

Two massive young men appeared, Christophe and Daniel Cabral. Mark Stover, Elias's son, a six-footer himself, stood unseen behind them.

Christophe spoke. "Mom said Stove mentioned Ben. Ben means trouble. We have to bring the old goat home in one piece."

Dowling shook his head. "Get these damn kids out of here!"

"Daniel just got back from basic training," Christophe shot back. "You fight with him. And where he goes, I go."

Daniel just nodded. Stover and Annibal were like uncles to one another's children. Stover put a calming hand on Cabral's shoulder.

"OK. I know better than to argue with a Cabral," said Ben. "We have limited resources. Deployment is everything. Lookouts will be crucial to our operations. We'll be counting on you."

"Yes sir." All three spoke as one.

Stover suddenly realized that Mark was hidden behind the enormous Cabrals.

"Oh, no!"

Stover caught Annibal's eye, and saw his friend nod with shared exasperation. *Not yet, Lord Jesus! Not yet!* prayed Cabral, knowing Stover felt the same. For once, the eloquent minister and politician stood speechless.

Finally, he stared hard at Daniel Cabral.

"Daniel. Keep your kid brothers safe."

"You got it, sir! But can't you find a better babysitter?"

"No. I can't. I'm trusting you, Daniel. I'm trusting you." Before he choked up, Stover turned back to the men.

"Go on, Ben."

"Daniel and Christophe and … and Mark can keep an eye on their two boats from a distance. From *Os Lusiadas*. It must be recon at a distance. If you arouse suspicion, no matter how good you are, they probably have toys that could ruin your day before you get a chance to be big and bad. You have to keep us posted. If communications are out, you may have to send someone back by skiff. Not Mark! He hasn't grown up on the water. If they bug out, shadow at a mile's distance and broadcast to the Coast Guard.

"For the rest of us, we may want to set up a zone defense kind of surveillance that becomes sort of like a mobile trap-line. There are no really good elevated vantage points except church steeples and lighthouses, the first places they'll look if they think there's a reception party. So, let's see if we can maneuver them into a trap or two along the way. We'll collect them one or two at a time, avoiding firefights and lethal force as best we can. First, like I said, they may be gas-lighted good guys. Second, we'd be outgunned in any firefight. Third, the island's full of tourists and locals we can't protect unless we present these guys with Peter, Eve, and yours truly on a platter. Fourth, we have no way to alert civilians without causing complete chaos. Plus the chief says major roads are messed up.

"We may just be able to get this done without creating a three-ring circus if we understand ourselves as guerrillas trying to cripple and capture rather than kill an invading force.

"Before you tell me I'm crazy, remember they want to reacquire Peter Souza and protect their operation. They're really here for extraction and damage control, not combat. They want to slip in and out unnoticed. If we can isolate and trap them, things may get nasty, but we probably can minimize risk to civilians.

"Phones seem to be down. We'll do our best with short-range cop radios, even knowing they may listen in. Remember, they can't move as a group until they locate their targets. We can use that against them. We'll spread out. If we identify folks, surround them in force and take them down without firefights, we'll whittle down a force we couldn't face head on.

"They have pictures of Peter Souza, and probably of Eve Gilchrist and me. I doubt Johnson would recognize Ray. We can't put Eve at risk. I'm best qualified as bait or to operate solo so I don't attract attention to any of the rest of you and compromise your ability to catch them by surprise.

"We have to assume they're all well trained. But for what? Doubtful they're accustomed to working as a large team. They may not know one another. Some were trained exactly like our two composers, but some probably went to badass school somewhere else and might throw us a curve. Absent reports of female operatives, we'll focus on suspicious males.

"What would make someone a suspect? Normal guys walk around either doing something and turning around, or, if they're just tourists, looking at the sites and stuff in shops, and checking out the women. The people we're looking for will be searching. There's a lot at stake. Maybe some clock we don't know about is ticking.

"They're young—probably combat savvy, spy-craft weak, hopefully too focused to be subtle. The kind of guy we're looking for will make a pretense of looking around. He'll stare at things that relate to their mission, but may make no sense to us. If they suspect we're looking for them, they'll scan every high elevation assuming sentinels could be posted there. Look for people looking up. They may put some of their folks up high. If so, we watch them and figure from their actions what they see and what they want to do. If they're scanning for a person, they'll check out what they think might draw that person, and what places have what draws them. For example, if Eve Gilchrist is a target, they'll have to check out every boutique and jeweler."

"Sexist!" muttered Rat.

"She's a beauty drawn to beauty," said Lucco. "Take Ben seriously. And Ben, no window shopping for fishing shit!"

"I'm not convinced Johnson would recognize Ray," Ben continued. "If he does recognize him, he'll know something's going on. In any case, Ray's immobile and must be kept safe. I don't know how to cover for Brazzo, Pacella, and Tomaselli. Johnson probably could finger them, and others will make two of you as cops.

"Rat, you'll be our cavalry. Ride a circuit and report in. We need your mobility. Me, maybe I can let them see me and draw a few into an ambush. The rest of you take streets and scout from inland to the harbor. Up and down, then one over. When you reach the end of the grid I'm marking on these street maps, go to the other end and repeat. Those who take the streets parallel to the water, same deal. When you make an ID, or suspect one, keep your eyes on the suspect. Someone else will be along. If you're rushed, use the radios or go to the corner of one of the streets that crosses yours. Someone will come along and help or carry the word."

"They'll be looking for Joe/Nick/Pete, and probably for Eve and for me. They may stake out Pete's family and friends, and wait for him to show. We'd like to get there first. But I'm still stumped about how to figure Pete's moves."

"Best guess?" asked Lucco Brazzo.

"If you were Pete wanting to find yourself, you'd probably go for your friends, your family, and Coach Mack. If you were Pete programmed to make your break with your past irrevocable, you might be sent to destroy, or figure out how to destroy, those very same people. So we need to keep an eye on them."

Pacella broke in. "OK. A lot of this shit I don't pretend to get. But I've raised a bunch of kids, and you may be missing your best bet."

"What do you mean?"

"Well, if you were an alienated kid, not sure if your family was your family and your coach was your coach, all of them would be like some kind of authority you weren't sure you could trust. Right?"

Everyone was listening now.

"So, where would you go?"

Ben nodded.

"Miserable young men either get smashed or try to go to the women they love. Maybe they hope to find salvation in their love, maybe … the rest is over my head. Did Pete Souza have a girlfriend here?"

"Nice," said Rat. "Much too smart for a cop."

"Good point!" Ben resumed. "I met her. He's already seen her and hurt her beyond words. But he may flip and behave like you say. I'll check on her."

Pacella reminded him, "Protect her too well and she loses her value as a person to bring Peter home."

"Damned if I know how to play that one, Tony," said Ben.

Tomaselli actually raised his hand. Pacella goaded him.

"Please, teach! Let him go to the little boy's room."

"I'm serious, guys. You know, I been thinkin'. And yeah, I'm not the brightest guy in the world. But that's a lot of manpower for one undergraduate."

Lucco Brazzo asked, "You talkin' economy of scale?"

"If I knew what the fuck that was, I could answer you. Get out of my face, smart-ass. What I mean to say is that this is like bringing a nuke to a spat between grannies. It's too much. There's got to be more than one of these guys. Maybe they have a small group, or a bunch of small groups of them. Maybe like a couple of folks handle … well, less than six. This one guy goes sour and they have over twenty people good to go and knowing what this is all about? No fuckin' way! For just one guy and a couple of handlers, why move in platoon strength? We're talking about the tip of a pretty dirty iceberg."

He turned to Dowling. "No way this is legit. And no way it's really the feds. I've worked with them a few times. They don't move like this stateside."

Ben smiled. "Well, the Philly PD is lookin' pretty good, notwithstanding its various affiliations. You make a lot of sense."

Stover nodded agreement.

"But let's use those various, that is, those allegedly various affiliations, effectively," Lucco suggested.

"I don't know about this!" Dowling growled.

"Listen to him, for God's sake!" Cabral broke in. "Whatever kind of smarts he has, you can bet the farm we don't."

"Listen." Lucco began, "Figure like this. Only for the sake of argument, imagine you're consulting a mobster that authorities can't catch and put away."

"We can fix that," said Dowling.

"Chief," said Lucco, "I know you're good people, so I'm gonna forget that awful thing you said. For shame!"

"I'm all ears, Lucco," said Rat.

"I like that even less," Dowling snarled.

"Don't get distracted, Lucco," Rat parried, "Dowling means well."

"OK," Lucco continued. "The problem is getting a group of heavily armed men past legitimate authorities in order to do what we will call a complex intervention."

"I don't believe that I'm listening to this crap!" Dowling fumed.

"OK, everybody but Chief Dowling, listen up. You want to hit somebody—say a Portuguese-American sleeper who's broken control, or a gorgeous doll and/or a worthless piece of shit I call my friend. But really smart cops know who you are and what you look like. Say they have probable cause to frisk you and ruin your day, and maybe your next few years to life.

"But that's just not on your wish list. So, you approach your target unarmed. But once you're past the cops you casually approach a van that just happens to have a fuckin' arsenal inside, pick up your piece, do what you have to do, dump it in the van, and do some chemistry on your way to a restaurant where your associates will swear you've been there all day. I bet that the white van, plus/minus the dark SUV, is for carrying weapons into town. Find their van, and cripple their plan. Then it's fist to fist. Knock down a few, cut them off from their weapons, and they may decide it's not their day."

"Lucco, that's pure genius! Prentice, if it's OK with you, Chief, I want you and every other volunteer you find or run in to out scouring this town for that van. Find it and report back. Rat, buzz the streets for the van before you take up your roving patrol."

Prentice looked to the chief. Dowling nodded, and added, "Before that, Prentice, tell the men watching the ferries to board and go to report the situation to authorities in Woods Hole and the Vineyard."

Rat wanted to be heard.

"I got two things to say. Then I promise I'll just shut up."

There were nods all around.

"I like Lucco's idea, and I've got one of my own," Rat said. "Kills two birds with one stone."

"Who the fuck are you?" came from both cops.

"Someone you don't want to meet in the dark. There are a lot of them and things could go down fast. You may want to neutralize a bunch to improve the odds. Now, seeing that I look so disreputable, and inspire so little immediate respect and admiration, and seeing that Signore Lucco over there can't pass as a choirboy, I have an idea ..."

As Rat explained his idea, ridicule gave way to shock, and then respect.

"If it comes to that, let's do it!" Ben agreed. "Chief, that play is yours to call. I like it the way Rat casts it, but we'll have to use whoever's available when things go down."

Dowling nodded. "Rat, who the hell were you in another life?"

Rat chuckled, and then became serious. "The second thing—if there are a bunch of guys like you and me that are still being fucked over in some a-hole military intelligence gig, nobody's war is over till we pull them out. Till then, their bodies may be home, but they're still missing in action."

"That works for me," said Ben. "Gentlemen, we stand adjourned for now. We'll use cop radios, even though they may be monitored. So, be careful. Check back at four if you haven't heard from me. You OK, Ray?"

"Yeah. I'm pretty immobile, though. Put me where I can help. If something goes down and you catch any of them, bring them to me. I want to talk to them."

"Why, Ray?"

"Cause Tomaselli and Rat got it right. Let me talk to them before you turn anybody over to Freddy Fed."

EIGHTY-SEVEN

Representative Elias Stover had a blinding headache. He excused himself, explained that he needed a few minutes to clear his mind, and walked away from the station.

Stover tried to see the world in simple, straightforward terms. The moral ambiguities of the situation he was grappling with were reducing his neatly organized rights and wrongs to shambles. After he left the SEALs, he followed his father to the pulpit, becoming a Baptist minister. Ministry led to community activism, politics, and in short order to the House, representing the urban, largely African-American community where he was born and raised.

To serve one master, Stover had lied to a man who deserved better. To further serve that master, he overrode the wisdom of his heart. He wanted to grab Mark, flee Nantucket, and get his son completely out of harm's way. But his friend and commander-in-chief, never expecting Stover would be endangered, had asked him to oversee this cursed situation.

He knew that Jordan's reports were congruent with information reviewed by his committee. If they were being dismissed, the stench of inappropriate influence was suffocating important truths. Elias and Ben were never close, but his SEAL team buddies Tomasso and Annibal stood behind Ben Jordan. At a gut level, SEAL to SEAL candor outweighed the intelligence apparatus of the federal government.

Stover wished he were confronting simple matters of right versus wrong. But this was treacherous moral terrain, two rights in contradiction. It was right to trust Jordan. It was right for him to follow the orders of his government. He couldn't force both into meaningful accord. Worse, it was an irrevocable fact that only a few short years before, Ben Jordan had put his own life on the line to rescue Stover.

Stover abruptly realized he'd walked too far while lost in thought. Turning back, he quickened his pace. Across the street, two young, fit, casually dressed men walked in the same direction. But they were walking a bit too fast, covering ground a bit too purposefully. Occasionally they stopped to look at something. Stover fell into step 100 feet behind them.

They stopped. One man put his hand to his ear while the other looked around. The first removed something from his ear, then reinserted it. He spoke to the second, who nodded. They resumed walking.

Stover was only fifty feet behind the pair on Main Street when the first man halted. Again, he raised a hand to his ear. *A bad connection*, Stover wondered, *or an ear bud that doesn't fit well*. The first cursed, "Fucking piece of shit!" His companion nodded in sympathy. *Could Jordan be right?* Neither seemed to be armed. *Could that mobster be right?*

The second man tapped the first on the shoulder, and pointed. Down the street stood a white van. As Stover walked past them, they crossed Main and took the next street to the left. He continued to the van. Peering inside, he saw nothing. He was turning away when another neatly dressed young man shoved him back against the van.

"What the hell are you doing?" he demanded.

"Nantucket Police. You want to see my ID?"

The man seemed confused.

"Sorry, man. I don't know what I was thinking."

"You sure you didn't just see a black man checking out your van and thought the worst? I could bust you for assaulting an officer of the law. But," Stover gave him a friendly grin, "I believe I'm talking with a good citizen who grew up in our still somewhat racist society. Am I right?"

"Yes sir! I feel like shit, Officer. I'm sorry."

"No problem." Stover turned to go, only to find that the two men he noticed earlier had come running up to the van.

"Hi, men!" he said. Looking back to the man who had confronted him, he said, "Well, I'll be moving on. Have a good day."

One of the two men who had just arrived was enraged.

"Who is this guy? What the hell was he doing? Why were you talking to him?"

"Relax. He's with the Nantucket Police, just checking out the van."

"Bullshit, you idiot!" the angry man hissed. He turned to Stover. "Who the hell are you? What the hell are you doing?" His companion popped the trunk of the car parked in front of the van.

"In there, asshole!"

Their attention focused on Stover, the three men failed to notice the stealthy approach of a massive figure making its way to the far side of the car near the van.

Before they sensed his presence, a deep voice boomed, "All right, asshole!" Annibal Cabral picked up the man nearest the trunk and threw him in headfirst, slamming the trunk's lid closed. With a lightning leap, he grabbed another, threw him to the ground, and smashed his head on the pavement.

Stover doubled his man over with a kick to the gut and put him down with a hammer fist to the neck. Cabral produced plastic ties for the two men they'd disabled. He fished keys out of their pockets and opened the trunk. A single punch convinced the man within to submit without further protest.

The two SEALs drove to the police station on Water Street with three unhappy men in the trunk.

"Fucking Jordan!" muttered Stover.

"Your language surprises me, Elias."

"He said you'd stick around and cover my six."

"Hey, what are friends for?"

"I'm blessed. We've got to call Washington and get some back-up. I hate it that Lucco Brazzo was right. He troubles me."

"I'm glad he's on our side."

EIGHTY-EIGHT

Chief Dowling sized up the three prisoners.

"Well, gentlemen. What do you have to say for yourselves?"

The man who'd threatened Stover snarled,

"I can hardly wait to see you and your jerk-off assholes fired and charged with obstructing federal officers acting in the line of duty."

"Congressman? Did these gentlemen identify themselves as federal agents?"

"No."

"Congressman, did they identify themselves as the representatives of any law enforcement agency, or indicate that they were involved in matters of national security?"

"No."

"How did they announce themselves?"

"This gentleman opened the trunk and said, 'In there, asshole.'"

Chief Dowling looked the men up and down.

"So, what the hell are you gonna do, dickhead?" The aggressive man sneered.

"I'm going to read you your Miranda rights, and take you into custody for assaulting an official of the American government, and hurting the feelings of the chief of police."

"But we're carrying out an assignment for the …"

"Shut up!" another of the men interrupted. "Sit tight. Our people will be here. Don't make things worse."

"Gentlemen, you have the right …"

Meanwhile, Stover had gone into another office to telephone Washington. He waited until the Miranda rights had been read.

"Chief. Your line is still dead."

The three men knew something. They kept smirking.

"Ah, I guess we'll have to add vandalism charges as well."

"Fuck you."

"Please talk to me now or you'll be incarcerated in a very special cell."

There was silence.

"Preston, conduct these men to a very special cell."

"Yes, sir! Would one of you gentlemen assist me?"

Cabral and James marched the three men out.

When Cabral returned a few minutes later, he was shaking his head in amusement.

"What's funny, Cabral?" asked Dowling.

"The hold of a fishing boat?"

"Strategy, Captain Cabral. If we keep everyone here and their buddies spring them, they're at full force and we have no evidence. If we disperse them, they can't regroup that easily. Odds are some will be available for interrogation. Seems to me that since they've cut us off from reinforcements, Jordan's idea of whittling them down sounds pretty good. Nicolai, would you believe, managed to corral a couple. He took one out, put on the guy's shirt, walked up to another and waved down our Philly cops at an intersection. Ray's watching them in a vacant store nearby."

Prentice James returned.

"Sorry, Chief. That white van belongs to a cleaning service."

"Of course," Dowling grumbled. "Why should things be easy?"

EIGHTY-NINE

Rat walked back to Ray's outpost. Ray's wounds continued to seep. Rat squashed the urge to badger Ray about medical attention. Realizing Ray's loyalties would drive him until he dropped or the battle was over, Rat brought him a Coke. Moving away from the prisoners, they spoke softly.

"Well, it's time for us weenies to head for the sidelines. They're sending out messengers and an SOS to the Coast Guard. Soon we'll see the real CIA."

Ray spat.

"Looks like you love the company as much as I do," said Rat.

"Probably more."

"Those bastards had some slopes on a chopper, taking them for interrogation. They asked one a question. He knew enough English to say 'Fuck you!' The CIA type didn't even raise his voice. He ordered this Marine to throw him out the hatch. Then, he asked the second slope the same question."

"I'm getting a real bad feeling."

"Yeah. Mr. CIA had a pearl-handled revolver pointed at my nuts. If I had any soul left, that destroyed it."

"You did the smart thing."

"The coward's thing."

"I was in a chopper once. Something like that went down. I said no. The guy said, 'OK' in a nice quiet voice, and put me under arrest. They tied my hands behind my back, tied my legs …"

"And then?"

"They threw me out of the chopper." Ray felt himself choking up. "No more."

"I wish I didn't believe you."

A minute of silence passed. Then Rat spoke.

"You'll understand. I keep my in-country name to remind me of the day I died. Yeah, I did some tunnel ratting. But that day they made me a different kind of rat. A dead rat. I just haven't fallen over. What did they call you in country?"

Ray turned to Rat. He had known many tunnel rats, brave men who fought terrifying underground battles in networks of underground passages the Viet Cong constructed. Some came away so traumatized they felt they'd joined the legions of the living dead. Ray gave Rat a vicious snarling smile. "Those who knew me best? After that day, they called me 'Big Chief Asshole.'"

Both men chuckled softly as they sipped their Cokes.

"The guy who threw me out … He saw this medicine bag, an amulet with a feather that I wore with my dog tags. Pulled it off my neck, said I wouldn't need it any more … And then it was time to fly. Air CIA!"

"Motherfucker!"

"Not my best day."

"I'll be back, brother. They want me to ride circuit and see what I can see."

"I'll stick around and practice for the triathlon."

NINETY

The boys grumbled down to the harbor and bitched throughout their Zodiac ride to *Os Lusiadas*. A small boat sped away from the harbor into the bay.

"Someone's got a lot of gas money," said Christophe.

Daniel barked orders, "Get on the horn, Chris! Mark, stand by to cast off on my signal."

"Hey, Daniel! No power, man!"

The Cabrals began to go over *Os Lusiadas*. Mark heard a fusillade of cursing in Portuguese.

"What's going on?"

"Somebody sabotaged our boat," said Christoph.

NINETY-ONE

Dowling took the news philosophically. He asked the Cabral boys to cruise the harbor in their Zodiac and find someone willing to transmit their message for help. Then he turned to Mark. "Son, these fellas know boats. They may bump into somebody they know. You don't have their savvy. No offense, but I think you have to step to the sidelines for now."

"Isn't there anything I can do?"

"I don't think so, Mark."

Mark left, but turned right back.

"Chief Dowling, I'm almost an Eagle Scout. I had to learn Morse code and semaphore flags. Let me try to send a message."

"Good idea!" *Might as well put a message in a bottle. No one remembers semaphores.*

Dowling wrote a message for Mark to transmit, and sent him far away from everything. He'd be occupied and safe.

NINETY-TWO

Ray sat in the storefront with two captured men in front of him, tied to chairs side by side. They wouldn't talk.

An athletic six-footer walked into the room slowly, even arrogantly. He wore a ski mask. He carried a half dozen baseball bats.

"Who the hell are you?"

The man said nothing. He walked out and returned with two tall stools. Walking out again, he came back with several heavy glass vases. He placed a stool alongside each man.

"OK, shit for brains number one and number two."

The men snickered and shouted obscenities.

"We're working together," the man said, "so I'll forgive those remarks. Now listen to me."

The man slowly took a batter's stance with a light-colored bat and splintered the front left leg of the chair holding the captive on the right, then the front right leg of the chair to the left. Only the pressure of their bodies against one another kept them from falling.

He positioned a heavy vase on each stool.

"Now listen to me." Inwardly the man reminded himself, *Maple bats first, ash bats later.*

Ray sat stunned. The masked man's voice seemed strangely familiar.

"Now listen to me," said the man. The voice. Where had he heard that voice? *Bobby Gray?*

With a great show of deliberation, the man selected a maple bat.

Ray jumped in, "Don't piss him off. I've got a weak stomach."

"And I've got a shit temper!" With one swing, the maple bat cracked through the legs of Ray's chair. Ray landed hard. A long, almost sword-like shard remained with the bat's handle.

"Damn you! Help me up."

The man pressed the shard against Ray's throat and drew blood.

"Maybe later."

He threw the shattered handle at Ray.

"Shut the fuck up."

He turned to the two men. "You listen to me, maybe I listen to you. This and only this is your meditation: How do you want to wake up tomorrow?"

The men laughed.

The masked man selected another maple bat. He took a practice swing. Both men winced. His next swing demolished the vase on the stool to the left. Both men cowered, shocked and lacerated by the shattered glass. One screamed as the sweet spot of the broken maple bat flew into his nose. The other howled when the masked man hurled the broken shaft at his head, and didn't miss. Both men bled.

He picked up the third and last maple bat, and walked to the second stool and vase. He took a practice swing.

As he drew the bat back, one man cried, "Wait! What do you want?"

"Where are they?"

"Where are who?"

"Listen to me." Again he swung. Again both vase and bat shattered.

"Shit. That half tore off my ear."

"Half doesn't count," said the masked man.

The second man stared at the remaining bats. He looked up at his tormentor.

"I see what's coming. It's not worth it. What are you offering?"

"I'm not."

The first man looked at the second. "He's bluffing."

The second stared hard at the masked man.

"No, I don't think so. I heard about this. It starts with the maple bats. They shatter easy. The ones he has left are white ash. Even if they break, his swing follows through and your brains get scrambled. I don't want to live that way."

"They'll kill us if we tell."

"That's some tomorrow God knows when. Today is today. I want to see tomorrow."

"I'll make it easier," the masked man said to the first captive. "Now! Or you can watch your more intelligent friend's head smash like a rotten pumpkin."

The second man vomited. He looked hard at his companion, the masked man, and at Ray.

"Nick G. is Joe Morgan at the U. Nick C. is Henry Gentry at Penn State. Nick W. is Jesus Mendez at the University of Delaware."

The man took a few practice swings, slowly and casually. His appearance of nonchalant indifference was chilling.

"50 percent isn't a passing grade, pumpkin head. Hope you like pain."

The first man broke in, "How the hell did you know about that? Sorry—never mind. They know. Let's live and hope that our guys pull us out of this.

"You're looking for the handlers that report to Johnson. They don't report directly. I don't know the middleman. But

Joe Morgan's handler is Marty Franks, posing as an undergrad. Henry Gentry's is Mahesh Mukarji, a graduate student in psychology at Penn State. Jesus Mendez is handled by Howard Wein, a grad student in psychology at Delaware."

The masked man nodded. "Shelf life?" he asked.

The first man answered, "I don't know. Whenever you ask, Johnson just chuckles and yawns."

"What does that mean?"

"As long as you have that bat, I wish I knew. I'm not afraid of dying. But I can't face being some brain-dead cripple."

The second man broke in. "Shit! He'll figure it out in five minutes and trash our asses. Tell him!"

The first cursed, "Well, I really didn't know. How fucked is that?"

The masked man laughed. He stage whispered to the first man, "You really want to tell me they are sleepers. Long-term, I assume."

"You got it," said the second man. "You got it."

"Gentlemen. You never want to see me again. Best chance for that is to exercise your intelligence and realize I was never here. Know that in your heart and soul. Asshole on the floor made you give it up. That's your story and you damn well better stick to it."

The masked man helped Ray onto another chair, none too gently. He checked the ropes confining the prisoners, tightened some knots, slapped Ray hard on the back of the head, and walked out.

NINETY-THREE

Prentice James passed the word about the Program's operatives and van to every volunteer or summer cop he encountered. Privately, he worried and prayed. *A white van? There are at least two dozen white vans on the island, maybe more. Lord, just give me a chance!*

Scouring Nantucket Harbor, Prentice already had checked out three white vans. *There was another, just ahead.* A man was walking away from it. *That's the same kind of shirt the others wore, but his is red! My God! Is that the van?*

Prentice watched as another red-shirted man come up to the van, opened a door, tucked a package into a gym bag, and walked away.

My God! This could be the one!

NINETY-FOUR

Steve Hamner was Johnson's second in command. He shared General George S. Patton's conviction that commanders should demonstrate to their troops that they too were soldiers and shared their danger. Accordingly, he carried a conspicuous sidearm, a commemorative reissue of his hero's pearl-handled 1873 model Colt .45 revolver. His windbreaker concealed his holster as he walked a circuit passing several places where Johnson anticipated Peter Souza might be found, out to a beach, and back. When a target had been located, he would rush to that location. Ben had given Rat a similar role—roving, reporting, and running like hell if needed in some particular place.

Looking toward the water for a moment, Hamner noticed flashes of color out on the bay. Focusing his binoculars, he made out several colorful spinnaker sails, ballooned out and close to one another. *Probably racing.*

Then some colorful flashes toward the shore caught his eye. *Kids flying kites*? He focused carefully. A slender African-American teen came into view, a colored flag in each hand. *What's that crazy kid up to?*

He pocketed the binoculars and began to walk off. A few moments later, something in the back of his mind began to bother him. Then it came to him: *Could that be? No! It couldn't!* But he had to be sure.

Hamner turned back, trying to keep a casual pace. Refocusing on the boy, he tried to remember something he'd learned years before. He'd forgotten a lot, but he recognized some crucial letters. *He's sending an SOS!* The boy was alternating semaphored messages with raising both arms and crossing and uncrossing them over his head, an international distress symbol.

Damn! He's calling for help! Representative Stover's son was with him on vacation! *Is that his kid?*

Hamner noticed a flashing light on a powerboat off shore. *Shit! Someone's responding in Morse code!*

Hamner walked toward the boy. Studying the boat's flashing light, he made out "a—s—s—i." The boat was either offering assistance or asking the boy if he needed assistance. Hamner began to jog. The boat altered course and sped toward the boy. Hamner broke into a run.

NINETY-FIVE

Ambassador Gilchrist loved to be the center of attention, but he listened to Buck with unwavering attention, asking few questions.

"That's all I know," Buck concluded.

They walked out past the bar counter, where Noah stood polishing glassware for the happy hour and beyond. Several crystal decanters and bottles rested on the bar, awaiting their turns.

Three men entered the bar and headed toward Ambassador Gilchrist. They stopped a few feet away.

"You'll have to come with us, sir," said their leader. "We don't want to create an embarrassing scene."

"I'm sorry, son. What did you say your name was?"

"I didn't. Please come with us."

"Slow down, son. Provide me with your credentials, or I don't budge."

Ambassador Gilchrist turned to the barkeep.

"What's your name, son?"

"Noah, sir."

"Well, Noah, would you please call the chief of police and let him know that three unidentified Caucasian males are here, apparently impersonating federal officers?"

Noah started to raise the telephone receiver.

Turning to their leader, the ambassador said, "I have no reason to believe that you have any legitimate authority. Perhaps you'll identify yourselves to the chief of police and we can work this out."

The leader turned to the others, "Take him. And this other clown, too, if he gives you trouble."

Buck caught Ambassador Gilchrist's eye. "If it comes to it—Freddy's."

"What does that mean?" The leader shook his head and stepped back to let the others take Gilchrist. Turning toward Buck he met an enormous fist that dropped him to the floor. The ambassador grabbed two heavy pitchers, smashed them against the bar, and slashed at the others. One went down at once, blinded by blood flooding down his lacerated forehead. The ambassador hacked at the second until the man was staggering, unable to defend himself.

"Enough, Mr. Ambassador. We don't need to kill him."

"Freddy's," said Ambassador Gilchrist.

Long ago and far away, the ambassador had been on a colossal bender, hiding out in a dive called "Freddy's." When Buck found him, thugs were trying to steal his wallet. Buck courteously asked them to leave the poor man alone. They declined. Buck smashed a pitcher and a bottle of cheap vodka, neutralized them, and toted Ambassador Gilchrist home in a fireman's carry.

Noah stood paralyzed, the telephone in his hand.

"Noah! The man said, 'Call Chief Dowling,'" Buck growled. "The show is over. What are you waiting for?"

"The phone is dead."

"Send someone! Unless you want this guy to bleed out on your floor."

NINETY-SIX

When he first spied a boy on shore waving flags, Rear Admiral Jed Marshall, USN Retired, waved back and resumed overseeing his son's often-erratic boat-handling. But when he looked back and saw the boy was still waving to no one in particular, he pulled out his binoculars.

Son of a gun! Is he just waving a flag? No! Two flags! The worst semaphore work I've ever seen! If a seaman on one of my ships ... The admiral hadn't read semaphore signals in years. *Just for the hell of it, what is that damn kid trying to say?*

Admiral Marshall leapt from his chair.

"Attention at the helm, Son! Slow to five knots. Prepare to alter course." He grabbed a detachable light he used for night-time landings and unlit anchorages. In Morse code, he made to the boy, "State is this real emergency. State is assistance needed."

As the boy began to respond, the admiral saw a man jogging toward him from behind. "Son! Come about and make for that boy with the flags!"

As his boat came about the man broke into a run. "Make full speed!"

"Aye, aye, sir."

"Everyone! That kid is sending an 'SOS.' Nantucket Police requests transmit to Coast Guard—armed men intruding—communications cut—inform CIA and FBI.' Mom, make that transmission! Boys, find whatever you can, just in case. Break out the flare guns. Our duck guns too. We may have to rescue that kid."

NINETY-SEVEN

Prentice James needed a plan. Shielding his eyes from the window's glare and reflections, Prentice made out some clips on the floor behind the seats, scattered among the golf equipment. This had to be van that was bringing Program operatives a small arsenal while his own Nantucket PD was locked out of its own armory, its locksmith nowhere to be found. Junior had tied up the locksmith in the man's own camper, where he would not be found before nightfall.

Prentice James knew he had to act. A surprising idea formed itself in his mind. The owner of the last van he'd checked was a friend. He let Prentice borrow his van and tools. Prentice rushed back to the weapons van with the tools and the second van's plates. He removed the plates from the weapons van, and mounted the borrowed van's plates in their place. The borrowed van had a dent on the driver's side door. Prentice made a ferocious kick that rendered both vans identical.

Then, he ran to his friend's van with the weapon van's plates and installed them. He sprinted a block to The Scrimshaw Duck, where he worked part-time as a waiter, and burst into the kitchen.

"Some real bad men are in town. They expect to pick up guns from a white van. I switched its plates. When they come, I want to arrest them and take them off the street. But the gun-carrying real policemen are nowhere near. I need some men to help me contain them. If I'm right, they won't be armed. If they run into a lot of men with knives and sticks I think we can hold them until help comes. If I'm wrong and they're already armed, it could go bad. If anyone wants to help me, pick up the biggest knife you can find and follow me."

"Wait!" The imperious voice of François Lamonde, The Scrimshaw Duck's flamboyantly gay executive chef, pierced the air. "What about dinner prep?"

"Chef, if these men start to shoot up the town, you can forget about opening tonight."

"Mr. James! Have you ever led men in battle?"

"No, Chef."

"Before I went my own way. I was an officer." François grabbed a flaming red boa from his gear.

"A captain!" He grabbed a jar of mustard. With a flourish, he painted two golden bars on each shoulder.

"*Mes amis!* Follow me!"

Like a deer transfixed by headlights, Prentice James stood momentarily immobilized as François led over a dozen waiters, cooks, busboys, and dishwashers out the door, every one wielding enormous cutlery. James recovered a fraction of his composure, and bolted after them.

What have I done? What have I done? Prentice felt transported into some surrealistic alternate reality as he ran to catch up with François and his damned red boa and his damned golden mustard captain's bars! *What have I done?*

NINETY-EIGHT

He had to silence that kid.

Hamner sprinted full out. Intent on his prey, he never looked back. He never saw a passer-by on a motorcycle brake to an abrupt halt. He never saw an unshaven man flanking him, bent low to the ground, a wrench in one hand, moving much faster than Hamner toward a point of interception.

Hamner threw Mark to the ground and drew his pearl-handled Colt.

"What the hell are you doing, kid? Who put you up to this? What did you send?"

Rat flew over the crest of a small dune, tackling Hamner from behind. Hamner lashed back with the Colt and struck Rat a glancing blow, but Rat controlled Hamner's gun hand. Grabbing his wrench from the sand, Rat ended their altercation with one powerful blow. He cuffed Hamner.

Mark handed Hamner's Colt to Rat. Rat's eyes grew wide. He could hardly move.

"Are you OK? Did you get hurt?"

Rat's eyes filled. He rested a hand on Mark's shoulder.

"I'm OK, Mark. Yes, I got hurt. But that was a million years ago."

Hamner opened his eyes to find his own gun pointed at his face.

"Kill the kid and let me go. Half a million cash! Work with me and I'll make you rich."

Rat fired into the sand near Hamner's head.

"I worked with you once. I didn't like the job and I didn't like the company."

"Who the hell are you?"

"Di du may!" Rat hissed. *"Di du may!"* He heard footsteps and turned. Three grim-faced men had come up from the beach. One was white haired, two thirty-something. They had seen Hamner menace Mark. They stared at him with undisguised contempt, their shotguns trained on his head.

"I haven't heard that since 'Nam," said the admiral.

"No, sir. Might you have some rope, sir?"

"Give the man our line, boys."

Rat bound Hamner securely.

"Did you get the signal, sir? Mark asked.

"Already received by the Coast Guard. Well done, son."

"What? What happened to the Cabrals?" Rat asked Mark.

"Somebody wrecked their boat. They couldn't transmit."

Rat turned to the admiral. "Thank you, sir. This is an unholy mess. Our boys didn't get through, but thanks to you and Mark, we may just stop some bad stuff dead in its tracks. I've got to get back."

"Can we be of any further help?"

"If you could transport this prisoner to Nantucket Harbor and deliver him to Chief of Police Dowling, and bring young Mark there as well, I would appreciate it. His dad is a congressman from Michigan, on assignment for the commander-in-chief."

"What's the story with this fella?"

Rat filled them in as best he could. Then he pulled out his badge and Miranda card, and shook Hamner.

"Mr. Hamner! As a deputized member of the Nantucket Police Force, I am about to read you your Miranda warning. Please listen carefully. You are going to be charged with a number of serious crimes. You have the right to remain silent. Anything that you say can and will be used against you in a court of law. You will have the right to consult with an attorney and you are entitled to have that attorney present during your questioning. If you are unable to afford an attorney, an attorney will be provided at no cost to represent you. In addition to current charges, you will be charged with atrocities and war crimes in connection with your actions in Southeast Asia during the American presence in Vietnam."

"How the hell do you know my name?" asked Hamner.

Rat held his face very close to Hamner's. "Back then I didn't have the balls to tell you I would never forget, that some day I'd come after you and do the right thing. But I told myself. Now I'm going to frisk you."

Rat confiscated a mariner's knife. In the zippered inside pocket of Hamner's windbreaker he found something unexpected. For a moment he felt faint and dizzy. Then he shook his head. It was hard to believe he was holding the object he now cradled gently in his hands. He took that thing as well.

"Anything else?" asked the admiral.

"Yes, sir. I don't encounter very many good men. I would like to know your name and have the honor of shaking your hand."

That accomplished, Rat gave the admiral a snappy salute.

"This young gentleman will fill you in on the way to Nantucket Harbor."

Rat turned, and walked back to his chopper.

"Dad. What did that biker say?"

"That former member of our armed forces and current deputy of the Nantucket Police? I'm sure I don't have to spell it out. Some day I'd like to sit down and spend some time with him."

NINETY-NINE

François called his restaurant workers to a halt a block from the van. He barked orders that left Prentice stunned and horrified.

"Think *West Side Story* without music! We'll come up on them like we're ready to rumble. Given our ethnic distribution, we are the Sharks. Every Hispanic, big vicious grin like you want to cut them real, real bad. Even if you're not Hispanic, play the stereotype for all it's worth. José? Pedrito? Grimace and scowl! See? That's what I want."

"Three or four of them are milling around," said James.

"How many should we expect?"

"I don't know. We'll let small groups assemble, like this one. I'll approach them. If things go bad, run. If not, wait for my signal."

François nodded. He held up his hand. His staff gathered around. "We divide forces now. Go left and assemble at the rear of the building behind the white van. Organize yourselves into two groups, one at each rear corner. Pedrito, you lead those on the left. Belle, you lead the people on the right. José, sneak up to be the lookout. I'll walk with you, Prentice. You're too contained, Prentice. I'll give the signal. I'll flip this red boa. *Mes amis*! When you come around, Sharks all the way. But if they have guns, cheetahs all the way—run like the wind! Go! Oh, Belle?"

Belle, François's diminutive Japanese sous-chef, looked back.

"Hispanic doesn't become you! Act like you once worked at Benihana!"

Belle cleaved the air with terrifying speed, smiled, and rejoined the others.

Prentice and François walked together as their band deployed.

Prentice stared at François in puzzled disbelief. "You?"

"Me, my straight-arrow African-American friend. You?"

"But I …"

"Enough, enough, Prentice. Don't mistake style for substance."

Six Program operatives drifted toward the van. One checked the license plates, nodded, and tried to unlock the van. His key didn't work. He re-checked the license plate and tried again.

When Prentice James and François Lamonde reached the van, they saw José was positioned perfectly.

"Gentlemen? A little trouble with your van?"

"We're alright," said one.

"Well, I hope that you won't mind coming down to the station with me. We need to talk with you about a number of things you may be able to help us understand more completely."

"That's ridiculous! Do you have a warrant?"

"Gentlemen, you are trying to enter a van you believe to be full of weapons. We have taken steps to block your access to its contents. You are under arrest for firearms violations, for conspiracy to commit violent acts, and many other charges as well. I will now read you your Miranda rights …"

"Don't listen to him!" another said. "He's not a real cop. He's just a volunteer. And this flaming faggot, whoever he is …"

François broke in calmly, "Gentlemen, we would prefer to conduct this matter in a civilized fashion, but …"

The second speaker shoved François, who deftly entrapped his hand and forearm. Bending the attacker's wrist, François forced the astonished man to his knees. He kept him subdued with one hand and produced a butcher's knife from behind his back. Everyone froze.

"Please, gentlemen. Don't mistake style for substance. Since I don't want to have to hurt anyone, and I assure you that I can, I renew our request that you come along to the station."

"Fuck you, faggot!"

François handed his knife to Preston and simply twisted the man's hand until he screamed with pain.

"That's Mr. Faggot to you." He shoved his attacker to the ground.

"Enough of your inadequacies. No more Mr. Nice Faggot!" François flipped the boa. His staff rushed out and surrounded the Program's men, paying faithful homage to a *West Side Story* frame of mind. Teeth and knives glittered in the sun.

"Gentlemen," said Prentice James, "Please obey Captain Lamonde's orders. And troops—if your prisoners misbehave, don't throw your knives. Just keep slashing till they can't stand."

ONE HUNDRED

Ben Jordan counted on being recognized and followed as he searched for Peter. He planned to lead his pursuers toward the patrol grids and maneuver for an intercept. Ideally, he would walk tails past his people, who could take them from behind. Shouldering his small knapsack, he started out optimistically.

His plan worked poorly, ensnaring only one operative. The Philly cops were moving in on another man when they saw Ben's signal. Tomaselli took down Ben's pursuer while Ben joined Pacella to capture the man the Philly cops identified. As Ben brought him to the ground with pressure point pain, passers-by took notice. But after Pacella cried out, "Dom! Dom! Didn't you take your insulin?" the interesting became mundane. The civilians moved along.

Ben walked slowly, strategizing. He waved to Maryellen, taking her children for ice cream. Rounding the next corner lost in thought, he almost bumped into Joe Morgan.

"Joe Morgan? I'm Dr. Jordan. This is the damnedest house call I've ever made. Maybe you didn't get my phone calls and letters."

Joe's confusion faded quickly. The guy who left his card!

"I bet you didn't think Student Health went this far out of state."

"This is crazy. What are you doing here?"

"I'm here to see if I can help you with your headaches, your fake names, your memory problems, and the crazy suggestions some asshole gave you that the woman you love is a slut."

"That's all beyond help. I've got to start all over again. Dr. Rivers told me so."

"Oh! Little Willie Puddle?" Ben sniffed the air. "The best thing about Nantucket is that I can't smell him from here."

"He said you and Gilchrist were dangerous."

"The only people I'm dangerous to are lying slimes like Rivers. The only people Gilchrist is dangerous to are envious other women."

"I can meet you halfway." Peter gave a wan smile. "But look, I guess you mean well, but I've tried to check out my past. I went back to my hometown. I tried to find my old friends and my coach. Hell, there's nobody in Somerset I remember, and no one who remembers me. I'm just fucked."

"You are fucked when it comes to Somerset."

"Shit! I'm not even in my team pictures!"

"Running back. Number 26. Right?"

"Yeah. How did you know that?"

"Stay with me. Your uniform colors ..."

"Hell! I got that fucked up too! I remember wearing blue and white, and the uniforms were actually dark blue."

"Got the name wrong, too, didn't you!"

"Yeah. I'm getting a headache."

"Bear with me. If I say 'Sean,' what do you feel?"

"Ow! It's getting worse."

"If I say 'Fletcher,' what happens?"

"Stop! I'm gonna pass out." Peter put his hands to his head. He sat down on the curb.

Ben joined him. "Bear with me. You were taught to feel lousy whenever you think of your best friend or your coach. Just picture your roommate for a moment."

"OK. That's better. What's going on?"

"Maybe you were conditioned to feel lousy whenever you think of people close to you. Let's try just two more. Hawkeye?"

"I thought I knew someone with that name."

"Linebacker?"

"No, quarterback."

"The one you threw that block for?"

"I used to think so."

"Bear with me. Merc?"

"Merc? Crazy guy. Tried to talk people into thinking that Mercury was the best car on the road. How do you know about him?"

"Well, I guess that whoever tried to brainwash you probably used some assessment instrument with statistical cut-off points, and didn't mess with anyone who fell below them. Sean and Coach Mack send their best, too."

"There was no Coach Mack. I went back to Somerset High. There never was a Coach Mack."

"Yes and no. There never was a Coach Mack at Somerset."

Ben paused. "But think for a moment. If Somerset was your hometown, why are we sitting in Nantucket? Why were you just screaming at your girlfriend on the beach in Nantucket where you two used to make out?

"A while back you went to Somerset. It tore you apart. But if you'd walked into Nantucket High instead, you would have seen that state championship trophy and team picture. There you are, wearing a blue Nantucket Whalers' jersey, number 26. The guy holding the trophy on one side is Coach Fletcher. Coach MacDonald Fletcher. You called him Coach Mack. The guy holding the trophy on the other side is your buddy Hawkeye Sims. Sean Fletcher is just behind you. And Merc is another row back on the left.

"That picture is just a few blocks away. Up for a walk?"

Peter's eyes filled with tears. He put his hands to his forehead.

"Ahh! What a killer!"

"At ease, Nick!" Ben rolled the dice again.

Peter shook his head. "It's calming down, but it's still a killer."

"Hawkeye was the team captain. He wanted to be a doctor. Remember? He took his nickname from that doctor on *MASH*. Coach Mack tells me Hawkeye's doing an OB-GYN residency in Seattle."

"Good for him! Merc?"

"Merc is assistant sales manager at a Ford dealership near Framingham."

"That figures! What have I been doing with my life?"

"You were in the army, and got selected for a rogue unit. You received prolonged intense training to carry out missions in an altered state of mind. They filled your mind with false memories and told you bad shit about the people you love to separate you from your past. Maryellen is no whore. Your brothers and sisters are alive. They live off-island. Your folks are OK, and so's your grandfather.

"I hate to throw so much at you so fast, but I don't want you to hurt Maryellen again, or mess up your future. Understand?"

Peter nodded. "Yeah. I know." He stood up abruptly.

"I don't know what you're doing to me. This is making me crazy." He started to walk away. When Ben started after him, Peter turned and cocked his fist. "Don't follow me."

I messed up! I tried to do too much too fast. I was so worried about Eve and Maryellen that I bungled my best shot. I probably made Peter feel I wanted to get to him just to protect them!

Ben was still berating himself when he ran into Lucco. He summarized his gaffe.

"I'm off to Nantucket High. I'll try again."

Lucco punched him in the arm, "That was just the first inning, my friend."

ONE-HUNDRED-ONE

Rat brought word that the Coast Guard had been called and Admiral Marshall was en route with Mark, a prisoner, and a functioning radio. He found the Cabrals and updated them about Mark.

When Christophe and Daniel learned about Mark's adventures, they were young enough to feel cheated rather than fortunate. Annibal shared their sense of futility. His first capture had been his only capture. The three Cabrals were primed to wreak vengeance for the attacks on Mark and *Os Lusiadas*.

The admiral let Ambassador Gilchrist use his radio. He repeated communications to the appropriate agencies, alerted the president, and contacted his wife.

"Betty, dear, we seem to have blundered into a very sticky situation." He summarized what he knew, and went on, "I believe *Cricket's Caper* is berthed near where their boats put in."

"I see the boats you described. Should I do anything?"

"No. The Coast Guard will handle it."

"The Coast Guard? I don't think so. So many boats calling in Maydays! They have their hands full."

"Don't identify yourself. That might give them ideas."

The ambassador repeated his wife's news.

Cabral spoke up. "They set fires all over the place on land to tie up the police and fire squads. I bet they sabotaged boats to mess up the Coasties. They trashed *Os Lusiadas!*"

Prentice James's crew dropped off their prisoners.

"Good work, James!" said Dowling.

"What next?" asked Cabral.

"What do you mean?"

"If someone with a weapon watched that go down, the next time around things might not go well. Are they waiting for you before they do anything?"

"I'm not sure."

"Rein 'em in, Prentice. Chief, I'm worried. We'll see what's going on."

"Take my .38."

"No, you hold the fort. Ben's afraid they'll try to break them out."

ONE-HUNDRED-TWO

Leaving the police station, Buchholtz noticed a tall, strongly built man in a red shirt trying to appear nonchalant. The man's jaw muscles grew tense as he watched other Program operatives being brought in and marched away. Buck walked past him, and recognized the bulge of a weapon in his rear waistband.

When asked about his time in the Marines, Buchholz would tell funny stories about tours in peaceful places. On embassy rosters as a guard, his main responsibilities were hidden in plain sight. He was often free to play with the embassy kids because his work was frequently nocturnal. "Sarge" was a plausible cover that described neither his rank nor his duties.

Buck sized up the situation, killed time until no one was looking, and subdued the man with ruthless efficiency. A woman carrying packages walked out of a store nearby as Buck knelt beside his adversary. "Damn!" he looked up to the woman. "Sorry about my language, ma'am. I just get so upset with him when he forgets his medicine and has these spells. I'll have to take him down to the hospital."

"Good luck!" she cried, "My dad is stubborn about his diabetes."

Buck pocketed Murdoch's ID and handgun. His rental car key tag gave its make, color, and license plate number. Murdoch was confined with ties in the car's trunk and transported to an old Boston Whaler, one of Dowling's creative holding cells.

Buck returned to the station. Efforts to deal with the detained and injured had spread into a nearby parking lot. An EMT was taking a break. He looked up at the big ex-Marine.

"Do you know what the hell is happening around here? I haven't seen anything this wild since a quiet day in New York City."

"Search me. I'm just a tourist."

"Right! Not with hands banged up like that. Jeez! There's a guy we took to the hospital. Two hundred stitches and counting. Did you do that?"

"No. Some other guy."

"What makes someone do something like that?"

"You threaten their daughter."

"Jeez!"

"Hey, long as we're talking, I have to track down a very pretty girl …"

"Don't we all?"

"Hell, no! Just marry a keeper! I'm looking for the gal whose father went ballistic. She's probably with a guy who'd be considered pretty good looking himself."

"Hmm! Both sort of tallish? She maybe five nine, five ten? Him six three or four?"

"Could be."

"They were walking toward Nantucket Cottage Hospital."

ONE-HUNDRED-THREE

Jim Cabot, "Dr. Gorgeous," was a senior resident in radiology at Harvard's fabled Massachusetts General Hospital. MGH specialists provided backup for the local hospital's small full-time staff.

Liam O'Shea, Cottage Hospital's radiologist, pursued his love of rugby long after he should have hung up his spikes, and finally paid the price. The best MGH could do at short notice was to ship over junior residents and give them vigorous support.

Jim's superiors at MGH appreciated his outstanding skills. When they learned he frequently spent weekends on Nantucket, he was asked to assist the junior residents by reviewing difficult films and diagnostic dilemmas.

Usually, Jim bore both this recognition and the extra duty it entailed with grace and good humor. But Maria Nunez, currently at Cottage, was a fretful bundle of nerves, indecision, and uncertainty.

Jim had just met Eve Gilchrist. Now, marching over to Cottage seemed an unreasonable imposition. He would have to tear himself away from one woman, who deranged his chemistry, to attempt the impossible with another—reassuring the perpetually panic-stricken Maria Nunez. Maria's anxieties threatened to devour precious time with Eve.

Jim was accustomed to dating exceptional women. Eve's looks, her self-evident wealth, and her brains failed to intimidate him. In ways Jim was unable to put into words, he was becoming infatuated and utterly fascinated at a pace he found deliriously intoxicating, downright frightening, and completely beyond his control.

They dined among the dunes on take-out lunches. They explored the island. Periodically Jim stopped at a pay phone. Sean was still involved in a nightmare case at Yale/New Haven.

"I have to drop in and review those films. Might as well get it done before Sean gets back. The gal who's on call is right up your alley. I'll try to make things quick, but I'm not optimistic."

"I'd like to come along. I don't see that many imaging studies these days."

Did I just say too much? Eve wondered. But she liked Jim's smiling response.

Jim and Maria Nunez reviewed a week's worth of studies. Maria had misgivings about many images. Like many psychiatrists of her era, Eve's first postgraduate year had been primarily medical. Films that puzzled and upset Maria held no mysteries for Eve.

"What about this one, Jim?"

Maria directed Jim's attention to a cluster of small calcified streaks, perhaps in a male patient's descending colon.

"I don't know, Maria."

"Do you think it might be some sort of teratoma?"

"Well, teratomas can include all sorts of tissue, including calcified elements," Jim reflected. "I'm not sure I know. But it's small, localized, and encapsulated, so whatever it is, it's probably benign."

Eve lost her self-control.

"Not for the gerbil!"

Jim studied the film closely with a magnifying glass.

"Yuck! Maria! Look over here. We misread those calcified areas, and there's something abnormal about the colon's lumen. With the magnifying glass you can actually make out the skeleton. Eve! How did you figure this out?"

"A celebrity in Philly went to an emergency ward when one got stuck. He had to explain it to the docs. Some members of the gay community insert a live gerbil inside some sort of plastic sleeve, and claim the rodent's death rigors are very stimulating."

"Is that the last one, Maria?"

"Yes, it is. Thanks, Jim. There's something I want to tell you. No. You can stay, Eve.

"Jim, you and many others have been very kind and supportive. But I've realized I'm not cut out for radiology. I need patient contact. I can't handle grinding through so many studies every day. I need time to think things through. Radiology is wrong for me."

"I'm sorry to hear that. But I understand what you're saying. What then?"

"Physical medicine and rehabilitation at a VA hospital back home in Texas. It's a better fit."

"It takes a lot of guts to face what you have to do and do it," said Eve.

"Thanks. And I hope the two of you will be very happy together."

Both Jim and Eve began to turn colors.

"Maria, Eve and I just met this morning."

"Jim, I may be slow about radiology, but I'm not slow about everything."

ONE-HUNDRED-FOUR

Ben had declined a weapon. It was a painful choice, but he was sure that when the enemy realized their men were being captured, they would try to break them out. He hoped his decision would not come back to haunt him.

He found Peter at Nantucket High, staring at the team picture, lost in a trance-like state.

"Hey, number 26!" Ben put down his knapsack.

"Oh, it's you. My head really hurts."

"I know. And I owe you an apology. I don't think I helped you back there."

"Looks like you were telling me the truth."

"Yeah, but I did it wrong."

"What do you mean?"

"I've been worried about Dr. Gilchrist's safety and I'd just met Maryellen Madeiros. Maybe they were too much in my mind when we spoke. I pushed you too hard, too fast."

"That's the Program."

"Whatever the Program is, that's not me. I should have been one hundred percent focused on you and worked at a pace you could handle. Like so many others, I gave you a headache instead of taking one away."

"That won't happen."

"Bullshit! With those headaches your mind and body are telling you that really toxic conflicts are tearing you apart. They probably said everybody like you gets headaches."

"How did you know that?"

"Because you can't feed people so much bullshit without their minds rebelling. They know your mind wants to defeat this crazy programming, so they teach you to stifle the healthy efforts your mind makes trying to reclaim itself. That leaves you open to being turned into some sort of super soldier, superspy, super whatever."

"How do I know that you're telling me the truth? I saw someone who looked like my grandfather walking over to the museum. But he must have been a fake. He's dead, isn't he? Or is he? I got such a headache!"

"Ask yourself … Now you know you've been told things that are false. You were taught those that you love the most are dead, no damn good, or impostors, right?"

"Yeah."

"But if they are dead, why are they also walking around, no damn good or not? Why are you so important that someone hired a whole fake Nantucket Harbor just to fuck you up? Doesn't that seem odd to you?"

"What do you mean?"

"Well, if you find they're alive, they're not really alive because they've been replaced by fakes or you're sure they're not who you thought they were. I bet that everybody was dead until you pushed back against your programming and went to Somerset that first time."

"You're right."

"But to me, the biggest proof you were conned is that mentioning Sean Fletcher gives you a headache, but mentioning Hawkeye or Merc does nothing."

"Why is that important?"

"Like I said before. Researchers follow the variables they consider significant and let other stuff fall to the side. They knew they should alienate you from your best friends, so they set traps to prevent you from reconnecting. But they didn't go after your whole circle of friends. You weren't as close to Hawkeye and Merc as you were to Sean. Will Rivers studied your life and followed the variables he found significant. Clinicians would want more detail, depth, and breadth."

"I must have been really mean to Maryellen. I think I hurt her this morning."

"You did, but she's crazy enough to love you anyway."

"I had a weird dream a couple nights ago."

"About her?"

"I don't know. Should I tell you?"

He automatically tells everything to the person in charge? Shit! I'll use it now and fix it later!

"Sure."

"It was complicated. First, this guy with a weird head was walking with some princess in Egypt. They wanted to have their own family. Then this Roman general was in some parade. He loved this noblewoman who loved him. Then, this Greek captain and his soldiers came home from battle. He ran to his family and wife, and they all collapsed on the ground hugging one another. All the women looked kind of the same, and sometimes I saw my face on these men. Somewhere in there was the word, 'Nerine.'"

"Jeez! I was afraid you'd give me a hard one! Whew!"

"That dream is easy?"

"Sure. Four years of medical school, four for internship and psych residency, a million more for analytic training and learning about hypnosis and dissociation, and it's easy."

"I guess I set you up for that."

"You can be my straight man any day. But here's how it breaks down. It combines Freud's ideas about the dream as wish fulfillment and Kohut's thinking about dreams that express the state of the self.

"In this dream, a man with many senses of himself, across those many senses of himself, is … Your turn to fill in the blank …"

"In love with the same woman. Egyptian princess, Roman patrician, Greek queen … They all looked so much alike."

"And they all were?"

"Maryellen Madeiros!"

"But Peter, the most important thing here is that at the deepest level, beyond whatever separate states you've been talked into, and no matter what they've been allowed to remember at a conscious level, all these guys in the dream—they are all the same man and they are all in love with the same woman."

"I hear talking inside my head."

"Let me help. Whether it's real multiple personality or the kind of thing that was done to you, no matter what you feel is separate, however strong your conviction, there's a deeper level still. At that level, you all are one. And at every level, you're being cheated out of the love of the woman you love. Let's suppose you've been made to experience aspects of yourself, organizations of yourself, as different. The basic strategy has been to get Peter Souza out of the way. Peter is just a nice guy, crazy in love with Maryellen. But he has skills someone thinks are useful. How to keep the skills and disconnect Peter Souza from what he loves? Convince him whoever he loves is gone! Once they're gone, why be Peter Souza? You can function better as Joe Morgan. How can you make Joe Morgan a first-rate operative yet keep him in plain sight, a sleeper as well as a man for special operations? Divide his awareness. Then, the question is how divided need he be?

"Maybe all you need is one more that Joe doesn't know about. But, what if the true core of Peter Souza keeps trying to emerge, what if Joe dreams of Maryellen and begins to put her face on every woman he's with? I guess they'd create one or more Mr. Insides to control the core of Peter Souza and keep the coast clear for that one Mr. Outside to come out and do the dirty work."

Peter seemed to have slipped into a trance.

"Mars is Mr. Outside."

"From your dream, I guess one Mr. Inside is Ares, the Greek god of war, or Odysseus, the returning warrior, and another might be the Egyptian fellow. Probably Set, or Seth. By the way, men ... I hope that while they were filling you with mythological names, they told you the name of the true consort of the god of war? They didn't! But in your dream, you knew, probably from those inside folks reading about themselves. Nerine, goddess of valor, is the true consort of all gods of war. You heard her name. Her manifestation in Maryellen Madeiros draws the warrior as well as the lover in you to her side. Protect her! Always!"

Peter nodded, still in trance. Ben heard noise nearby. Time was running out. From what Maryellen had said, Peter had to be exceptionally hypnotizable, off the scale hypnotizable. *Roll the dice again!*

"Shake my hand, Peter." Ben rushed into a crude version of Erickson's handshake induction. Shaking Peter's right hand with his own, his left hand slid under Peter's right. As he released Peter's hand, his left hand delivered a subtle upward push.

"And notice how your hand becomes lighter, it just seems to want to rise." He avoided metaphors of sleep, staying with the language of eyes-open waking hypnosis.

Peter's right arm rose as if an invisible helium balloon were pulling it skyward. His eyes were open, his face alert, surprised and amused. "It's just floating!"

Ben rolled the dice again. *I hope Mack and Philippe taught me enough!*

"I'm talking to the entire human being, to every identity that's yours by birth, by experience, and by training, across all names and times. Underneath everything is a solid young man, fucked over by people who played on his patriotism, his goodness of heart, and his hypnotizability. I talked to your grandpa, Philippe. He's an old sailor with an old sailor's ways of talking. I had to ask him to translate some of what he said 'cause I don't know Portuguese. He told me to tell you that that Michael Johnson is a ripe piece of goat shit, and that Will Rivers and his associates like Frank Brewer, Marty Franks, the whole bunch, are cow-cunts. He wonders ... Do you remember how to bait a lobster pot? Or mend a net? Or have you forgotten who you are. 'Peter Henry,' he asks, 'Prince Henry, are you lost at sea? Can you box the compass? Can you set your course home? Do you remember where we found the big ones?' He asked me to ask you that."

"Right off the point. Then we might sneak up the Childe River to get some mussels. Mom loves mussels."

"I know that place! Cove on the east side. Let the tide go out, and grab 'em just like that! Off the point for sea bass, into the cove for mussels, go home, crack a cold one, and feast! Your grandpa's the guy with that beat-up green and purple skiff."

"Yeah. The colors of the Portuguese flag. That's Grandpa!"

Footsteps grew closer. Ben's mind raced. Removing programing is difficult long-term work. If Will designed Peter's programs and activation codes, he'd use numbers. One item in the Stanford hypnosis scales instructs the subject to forget a number. Experimenters observe how subjects' minds develop irrational notions to explain their way around the missing number. *Go for it!*

"You were taught a number of codes."

"Yes."

"From now until this order is cancelled by me, the order of numbers is 1, 2, 4, 5, 6, 8, 9, 10. They are in sequence, in order. There are no other numbers below ten. Repeat."

"From now until this order is cancelled by you, the order of numbers is 1, 2, 4, 5, 6, 8, 9, 10. There are no other numbers below ten. Understood."

"Remember. Leave trance completely alert as I count from four to one. Four, two, one."

Too late! Armed men in red shirts approached. Three blue-shirts emerged from the gym door mere feet away.

One man had a bandage over his nose.

"Out of the hallway! Into the gym."

"God! I'm glad to see you, Nick! Welcome home!" Johnson pumped Peter's hand. Then he turned to Ben. "Jordan, you've been fucking with government research projects. He could be hurt if you don't back off."

"Really? I was thinking he might lose everything that's important in his life if I did that."

"Nick," said Johnson, "Execute B-3."

Joe's, Peter's, Nick's hands went to his forehead. Three no longer existed!

"Nick! Execute B-3!"

"Order not understood."

"Kill that man."

Peter punched Ben in the jaw, and immediately collapsed, his face contorted with confusion and horror.

"Nick! B-9." But 9 had lost two of its antecedents! 9 now was either 7 or 9 or 11 or something else, depending on how Peter's mind had read the warped command.

Peter rose from the floor, still dazed.

Ben screamed. "Nick! No more B numbers! Be Peter! Go to Nerine! Be Peter and don't look back!"

Peter raced away, knocking aside the blue-shirts as he ran.

"Red-shirts stay," Johnson ordered, "everyone else in pursuit!"

Johnson pointed to a chair in one corner of the gym. A man rushed to bring it over. Johnson crossed his legs casually, and appraised Jordan.

"Well, sometimes I hate to be right. I warned one of my men that you shouldn't be underestimated, and that he shouldn't use these idiotic robot command codes."

"Brains like yours and you delegate serious responsibility to Little Billy Puddle?"

"What can I say, Jordan? Good help is hard to find. I asked him if you could be turned. He said no."

"Yeah. If they had appreciated the quality of your work, not that I approve of it, or if Rivers were humane enough to give Joe stronger meds for his headaches, we wouldn't be having this charming conversation." *They haven't frisked me. If I can keep him talking …*

"True. And if you stuck with baseball, I'd be asking for your autograph. Yeah. I did my research. I won't insult you by trying to break you down. Take this as a compliment. You two! Drag Dr. Jordan out and kill him! Everyone else back on task."

A voice, behind Ben and to his right, barked, "Hands above your head!"

Ben felt a shove from his left. Both men were behind him.

All those years of breaking cinder blocks! Here we go!

Ben flung both arms back, smashing down the men behind him before blasting Johnson in the face. Turning back, one man was on the floor, the other staggering to his feet. Ben stomp-kicked the first and smashed the other's larynx. Johnson was already across the gym, shouting "Everyone back! Kill Jordan!"

Before Ben could grab a weapon, someone thrust a sub-machine gun through the gym door, shooting blind. Ben ducked until the shooter stopped to change clips, and charged after Johnson.

ONE-HUNDRED-FIVE

A sharp ringing sound startled the men at the station. Chief Dowling smiled as he reached for the receiver.

"Thank God! We have our phones back." As he listened, saying little, he nodded to the others and gestured "thumbs up" several times.

Finally, Chief Dowling put down his telephone and looked up at Ambassador Gilchrist and Buck.

"Well, help will be here soon. NIS is lifting off from Newport in less than half an hour. Boston FBI has a team on the way to a helipad. The CIA won't say anything except that they are coming, the smug bastards. What a day! My own damn town! My own damn island! And I've been as useful as tits on a bull! You two put a bunch out of action yourselves."

"Buck deserves the credit, chief," the ambassador said. "You're our nerve center. Generals don't do privates' work."

Dowling's radio squawked. He listened and nodded. "That's one of my volunteers calling in. Some near-frantic bartender named Noah at The White Elephant, where all that went down? He says five more guys stopped by, looking for you or your daughter. They threatened him. He said you were brought here. They said they were coming to get you.

"Buck, take the ambassador and disappear. I'll hold the fort."

"You'll be a sitting duck alone here."

"Find Brazzo, Pacella, Tomaselli, or Rat—say Rat's plan is on. See five men. Rat's plan is on. See five men."

Buck and the ambassador left through a rear entrance. Chief Dowling appeared to involve himself in matters demanding his rapt attention. He seemed not to notice the man who walked past him into a cell, closed its door, lay down with his back to the chief, and began to snore loudly.

Minutes later five angry men appeared.

"We're here to take charge of Ambassador Gilchrist and ensure his safety."

"You boys feds?"

"Yes."

"Well, you know the drill …"

"Now!" screamed the man who seemed to be their leader. Veins stood out on his forehead. He was about to say more when he was distracted by a thunderous grating snore.

"What the fuck is that?"

"One of our regulars sleeping off a bender," said Dowling. "He's got some problem that makes him snore like that. I forget its name. Oh, yeah! Obstructive something."

"Obstructive apnea," one man said, "my uncle …"

The leader silenced him with a deadly glance.

"Boys, I'm glad to cooperate. This is not our kind of case. The guy sleeping it off is more our style. The ambassador? Yeah, we have him. And we hid him away real good.

"But rules are rules. Show me your ID. You look OK to me, but some FBI guy just radioed from DC. Not a happy man. Let's see. He said something like, 'Listen to me, you stupid son of a bitch! This is an FBI case. If you let some other people'—I guess that's you—'talk you into letting them take him away, we'll charge you with obstruction of justice and interfering with the activities of federal officers in the performance of their duties.'

"Tell you the truth, boys, I'm six months from retirement. I don't want to lose my pension. Let's do this by the book. Show me what I need to see. Then I'll put your big dog on the phone with me and some big dog from the Bureau and we'll work this out."

There was a knock on the door.

"Come in. We're having quite a coffee klatch."

Tomaselli and Pacella dragged Rat through the door. Rat's face was dirty. His shirt was torn. His hands appeared to be cuffed behind him.

"Who the hell is this?"

"This is the dirt-bag we talked about yesterday," said Tomaselli. They produced their badges. "Tomaselli and Pacella, Philadelphia PD. We've been chasing this a-hole for a year and a half. Sells his shit to little kids in South Philly."

"I didn't do a fuckin' thing, man," Rat whined. "You got me confused with somebody else!"

"Yeah! That's why we chased you all the way up fuckin' 95, with you carjacking some poor folks around Darien, and again at Westerly, and scaring decent people with your ugly mug all along the way."

"Cops scare me. I don't trust you guys."

Rat looked at the five men.

"Hey, man! Are you the feds? Let me surrender to you. These two'll kick the shit out of me the second you're gone."

Pacella shrugged.

"All these dirt-bags are the same." He mimicked Rat's whine, "I didn't do it. It must have been someone else. Your mama, it was someone else! Well, you guys were here first. We'll wait."

The five men joined in a chuckle.

"Actually," one said, "You may wait quite a while."

He pulled out a Walther PPK and pointed it at Pacella and Tomaselli.

"Frisk 'em!"

A man went over both. "They're not carrying!"

Pacella and Tomaselli shrugged. Pacella said, "We hit town and identified ourselves to Chief Dowling. He says we can't carry here. They're in his locker. Check for yourself. Great plan, Chief!"

The five snickered. "Yeah," one said, "I guess we could if some fuck hadn't welded it shut."

Tomaselli seemed to lose it completely.

"No fuckin' way! No fuckin" way! Dowling! Where the fuck are our pieces? We took this asshole down with our bare hands, but this is ridiculous!"

Rat began to whine about police brutality.

The leader of the five raged, "Shut that bastard up, you assholes, or I will!"

"I'll shut up! I'll shut up! Just don't hit me no more!" cried Rat. When the five men began to laugh, two automatics materialized from somewhere behind Rat's back and appeared in the hands of the Philly cops.

"There are five of us, asshole!"

"Yes," said Dowling, "and I see one Walther PPK."

"Go for it, Joe!" the frisker cried.

"Not so fast." The man who had appeared to be sleeping off a bad drunk pressed a shotgun to the leader's head. Rat produced Hamner's .45.

"Plan B! Hands up, douche-bags! Now!" said Lucco Brazzo. Soon Lucco's former jail cell housed five very enraged men whose connections with any federal agency remained to be clarified. Dowling found Rat some shells for the .45. Shaking his head, unable to believe what he was doing, Dowling handed the PPK to Lucco.

"Thanks, Chief. I'm OK. Give it to Prentice."

ONE-HUNDRED-SIX

Ben retrieved his knapsack and slipped into the vice principal's office. A man with a Heckler & Koch machine pistol backed into the room. Ben shoved the vice principal's chair into him and attacked. Soon he was bound and gagged in a closet. His weapon's clip was almost spent.

Ben heard two men approaching the room. The first started in, leading with his H & K. Ben grabbed its barrel and clubbed him with his comrade's weapon. The second shouted, "He's here!" and backed away.

Ben hooked an arm out the door and sprayed the hall. A voice screamed in pain. A body fell.

Glancing down the hall, one man was down, with more coming Ben's way. Ben grabbed the second H & K. Firing a burst in their direction, he sprinted across the hall and scrambled downstairs to the basement.

ONE-HUNDRED-SEVEN

"As long as we're here," said Jim, "I'll show you the rest of the joint."

They were walking down a basement corridor when a man held up his hand like a traffic cop and ordered them to stop.

"Excuse me!" said Jim. "I'm Dr. Cabot. You're not on staff here. What do you want?"

"Well, Dr. Cabot. I'm a federal agent, authorized to take a certain Dr. Eve Gilchrist into custody."

"Of what is Dr. Gilchrist accused? Let's see your identification."

"You have no right …"

"Yes, I do! Have you been cleared to enter patient areas? We have to be careful about nosocomial infections. Show me your clearance card and federal ID or get the hell out. We've been vaccinated against the unusual bacteria around this unit. Have you?"

The man hesitated for a moment, and then smiled.

"That's the best bullshit I've heard in years! But you shouldn't try it when you're standing in front of the door to the Housekeeping Department."

"I'll try to remember that," said Jim.

"Nice try, funny man. I'd kill you just for laughs. Dr. Gilchrist, you've got to come with me."

Jim turned to Eve.

"What is this about?"

"That case. People have been trying to get me."

"Now!" said the man.

Jim sized up a nearby maintenance cart.

"Yes, indeed. Now!" Shoving the cart into the man, he grabbed Eve's hand and pulled her along.

"Survival now. Talk later."

As they tore around a corner, the man was thirty feet behind and closing rapidly.

Jim guided Eve back to the Radiology Department.

"What are you going to do? Image him to death?"

"Something like that. Run!" Jim grabbed a small bag and a broom from another janitor's cart on the fly. Moments later, they closed and locked the MRI room's door behind them.

Signs screamed "All Metallic Objects Must Be Removed From Your Person Before Entering This Room." MRIs' powerful magnetic fields capture loose metal items and transform them into tiny missiles. Anything between them and the machine is in harm's way.

"Other side of the door. When I say run, get out of Dodge. You remember all about MRIs from when you were a real doctor?"

"You'll pay for that!"

Jim changed settings on the MRI's control panel and handed Eve every metal object he carried.

"When I make my move, duck low and scoot. Get to the police station."

"Oh, great! I meet an interesting guy and he calls me a fake doctor and plans to get himself killed." Eve gave him an impulsive kiss. "You won't get away with this!"

Two bullets shattered the lock. Jim positioned himself carefully. His body concealed the panel of switches on the wall behind him. In one hand he held a small paper bag by its bottom. The other grasped the broom behind his back.

Their pursuer entered the room cautiously, and turned slowly to stare at Jim, eye-ball to eye-ball. He pointed his gun at Jim's face.

"OK, laughing boy! What's behind your back? Nice and slow."

Jim threw the switches as he surrendered the broom.

Sounds came from the MRI machine.

"A broom. What were you gonna do? Fight me with that?"

"Not much else around here."

"Still the wise guy, eh?" Johnson's man drew back his gun hand to pistol-whip Jim.

"Now, Eve!"

The man barely glanced toward Eve as she ran.

"You first, her later." He never struck Jim. His arm's forward motion ground to a halt. He clung to his gun, but every molecule of metal in his weapon was caught by the inexorable power of the magnetic field.

Holding the paper bag by its bottom, Jim tossed its contents toward the man.

"Catch!"

Dozens of three-inch long ten-penny nails found the shortest distance between two points, heedless of the body in their path. Impaled by steel projectiles driving toward the very heart of a field that compelled every molecule of every nail to draw closer and closer, obedient to its pull, the man remained erect. He hung like a human pincushion surrounded by a growing lake of red, his face forever fixed in horrified surprise.

Jim turned off the MRI, taking the gun as the man collapsed to the floor.

Jim tied him where he fell with electrical cords. He scribbled a quick note: "Recalibrate before using. Dr. Cabot." Then Jim shoved the weapon into his waistband, pulled out his shirt to hide it from view, opened the door, and shouted to Eve.

"My God! What happened here?"

"Just another poor soul succumbing to the force of my magnetic personality."

ONE-HUNDRED-EIGHT

Mack found Buck near Main and Federal.

"Thank God, Sean finally got home! Just after I filled him in, Peter showed up. Sean picked up some tackle, bought some squid, and they jumped into one of the Souzas' skiffs. Peter was at the helm, grinning ear to ear."

"How's your health, Mack?"

"Hell of a question!"

"Answer it!"

"I can do anything I ask my kids to do. Just one hell of a lot slower."

"See that couple coming toward us?"

"Geez! That's Jim Cabot and Eve Gilchrist."

"Turn around and pull your cap down. See two guys behind them, gaining on them?"

"Yeah."

"We can't let them get the kids. If you're up to it, we're going to ruin their day. I'm taking them down, with or without you."

"Call the play."

* * *

Two large middle-aged men studied store windows until the young couple and their shadows had passed. Then they fell in behind the two men, gaining on them slowly and carefully. One took two beach umbrellas from a sidewalk display, handing off one to the other.

Coming up behind their targets, they thrust the umbrella shafts at an angle between their targets' legs, and pushed them forward, throwing them to the pavement. Two determined men who coached wrestling as well as football easily controlled their grounded adversaries.

A passer-by stopped.

"Any problem, Coach Mack?"

"Everything's under control. But could you run down to Josie's and get some rope, or even a few jump ropes? Tell her I'll drop by to settle up for them and these exceptionally sturdy beach umbrellas."

* * *

Soon two Program operatives were bound in pink plastic jump ropes with pink and white tassels on their handles. Josie relished being part of the excitement. She closed her store, drove everyone to the police station, and came home with a story she would embellish lovingly for the rest of her life.

ONE-HUNDRED-NINE

Annibal Cabral huddled with his sons.

"Nobody—nobody—gets away with messing with our boat." Cabral had purchased three items, now wrapped in brown paper, from a hardware store on Orange Street.

They circled the blocks where the decoy and weapons vans were parked. On their third circuit, a red-shirted man near a blue Blazer double-parked alongside the weapons van was shouting and waving to someone they couldn't see.

Annibal was beginning to size up the situation when he saw a blur of motion behind the red-shirt. Nicolai tackled him, kicked his weapon away, and began to punch him into oblivion. A second red-shirt left the white van to pull Nicolai off his comrade.

Annibal ran to help, but Daniel and Chistophe raced by him. Daniel knocked the second man out with a single blow to the neck and pulled Nicolai to his feet. The brothers tore the brown paper off two large axes. They were tying the men up with the men's own shoelaces when Annibal reached them.

"Nice work! You guys are scaring me. Let's check out the Blazer and van. We don't know what's inside."

A man trying to get out of the Blazer encountered Christophe with his raised ax and surrendered. The Blazer was empty. Annibal used his brand new sledgehammer to break a van window. He let himself in and found it was packed with weapons and explosives. Annibal was climbing out when he heard unwelcome sounds. *Ticking! I hate ticking!* Behind the front seats and under a blanket wires led to and from a small LED display that read 5:43, then 5:42, then 5:41.

Annibal shouted, "They activated a bomb." One man was out cold, and two seemed clueless. "Nicolai and Daniel, control them and hold the fort. Christoph, get help. I have to take a ride."

Annibal hot-wired the van and gunned it onto the sidewalk till he could swing back onto the street. He leaned on the horn and shouted warnings as he made for the harbor. When he slowed at an intersection, strong brown hands grasped the window frame.

"They told me! How much time?" asked Prentice.

"Four max! I'm going for the water."

They rounded a corner into a traffic jam. Annibal burned rubber in reverse and tried another street. Somehow Annibal and Prentice screamed, honked, and pushed through cars and crowds. The harbor lay just ahead.

Preston shouted, "Hey! If the crowds are here, probably the ferry just left. Head for Steamship Wharf!"

As they tore into the Steamship Authority's lot, they realized the ferry was departing late. It had just cleared the dock. Already cars were rushing into the lot, lining up for the next boat.

Annibal glanced at the timer—1:18! He braked. "Get off now!"

"I'm with you!"

"Now! Or I can't jump! Clear me a way!"

Cars and trucks and tourists! Annibal needed a clear shot to the water, but drivers eager to avoid delays at Woods Hole by boarding and disembarking first gave him no more than elevated middle fingers.

Two middle-aged women rushed screaming from the Steamship Authority office. "Stop that van! Stop that van!" Authority personnel came running toward Annibal.

0:32! Still more people coming! 0:30! Annibal saw no break in the circle of people and vehicles closing around him. Preston James drew the PPK and fired two shots skyward. "Hit the deck!" he screamed, "Police business! Out of his way! Out of his way!"

Frightened people hit the ground. Annibal made for a gap … The screaming women filled it at once.

"Bomb! Out of the way or I'll run you down!" He accelerated toward the water beyond the two incorrigible women. Prentice pointed at one. Annibal drove and Prentice sprinted right at her. Prentice pulled her to safety and Annibal jumped from the speeding van.

He rolled to a stop just before the end of the pier. The white van's brief, ungainly flight ended with a clumsy nose-dive. He wiped blood and grit from his face. For three or four seconds, there was complete silence. Then several loud explosions were followed by hundreds of small sharp reports from the clips of ammunition.

Prentice crawled up alongside Annibal. They watched the fireworks until everything was still. Finally, Annibal flopped on his back, exhausted.

"Prentice. I was so afraid someone would get hurt. So afraid." Cabral shed a few tears of relief, gathered himself, and struggled to his feet. Abrasions from his leap and roll left his clothing soaked with blood.

The angry woman Prentice had rescued rushed up to them.

"Officer! Arrest this man! He's terrified everyone! He disrupted our loading process! He drove that van right into the water! And you! How can you call yourself a policeman? You should be ashamed of yourself."

ONE-HUNDRED-TEN

Rat saw the NIS helicopter coming in. He raced to meet them and showed the men to the station. Then he tracked down Ray.

"It's a funny world, Ray. Too fuckin' funny."

"How do you mean?"

"Met an old friend a few minutes back. A-hole named Hamner. Had a great reunion. Loads of fun."

"Oh?"

Rat pulled the pear-handled revolver out of his waistband.

"It's a General Patton special. One I've seen before. Pointed at my nuts." He threw Ray a sailor's knife. "Spoils of war!"

"Are you shitting me? That's amazing."

"But that ain't the best part ..." Rat reached into his pocket and withdrew something with great care. He handed Ray a small leather bag on a torn leather thong, closed with a silver clasp with turquoise insets. The soiled stub of an eagle feather remained in the clasp.

Ray felt himself fading out. Somehow, he willed himself back from the brink.

No! How could this be? He was holding the very medicine pouch he'd carried as a younger man. A medicine man, his grandfather's friend, made it specifically for Ray and blessed it with long chants Ray barely understood. It was part of him until it was ripped from his neck by the man who shoved him out of a helicopter, bound hand and foot. The leather thong had been torn, and tied together with a crude square knot.

Ray felt sobs coming, far too powerful to control. Then Rat was holding him, saying "It's OK, buddy. It's OK," over and over till Ray could sob no more.

Ray caught his breath and struggled to find his voice, now little more than a harsh rasp.

"Where is he?"

"I tied him up with his head in a toilet. He's not going anywhere."

Ray pulled himself up. Rat looked questioningly toward Ray's wheelchair, then to his cane. Ray shook his head and forced himself to stand.

"Where is he?"

"Follow me." Protests would be futile.

In a men's room of a maintenance building nearby, Ray found Hamner, the man who tried to kill him. He was bound hand and foot, the ropes on his wrists tied to the ropes that bound his ankles. Rat had wrapped duct tape around his torso and neck and the back of the toilet, binding him head first into the bowl.

Rat flushed the toilet.

"Attention, you piece of shit!"

"Cut the tape."

"You sure?"

"Cut the fuckin' tape."

Rat sliced through the duct tape and pulled the man out of the toilet. He turned Hamner over and left him on the floor.

"When my men get here," Hamner snarled, "you'll wish you were dead."

"I've been wishing I was dead a long time," said Rat. "But I'm beginning to feel a little bit better."

The man saw Ray's medicine bag around his neck.

"Well, lookee here! The big bad Injun. I didn't know your name at the time, but hell, when I checked, I thought hawks could fly. What y'gonna do, Red Man? Scalp me? You're dog meat."

"Scalping? Hell, that was the white man's idea. You thought we were no better than animals. You got your bounty for killing us by bringing in a pelt of our skin and hair. I don't follow the path of the white man."

Ray's voice grew calm. "Who are you?"

"I'm the guy who's gonna watch my guys waste you any minute now. Payback will be a bitch!"

"Well, if we're in a rush, listen up! You are nothing!"

Ray looked around for suitable material. He shoved a wad of toilet paper and rags into the man's mouth.

"Those rags smell of gas," Rat said softly.

"Not enough," Ray saw a gas can among the equipment nearby. He poured a little gas directly onto the rags.

"Listen up! I am Ramon Two Hawks. My father is Mescalero Apache, of the Niitahende Band, the People Who Live Against the Mountains. My mother's people are Mexican Apaches and Navahos. I graduated from Arizona State and I was drafted while I was still a human being. You broke my back, but you could not break my spirit. I survived you and I will survive whatever you throw at us today, any day. In this world or the next, I will see you rot in hell.

"But first, a preview of coming attractions." Ray set the paper and rags afire. Hamner's eyes grew wide as saucers.

"Well, hot damn! There's a CIA man in trouble. Time for the noble red man to gallop over the hill to his rescue! Don't worry! I'll save you, Kemosabe!"

Ray unzipped his fly and began to urinate. As fluid ran down Hamner's face the flames were snuffed.

"Let it never be said that Ramon Two Hawks of the Mescalero Apaches so hated another living creature that he would not piss on him when he was burning."

"Let's go," Rat urged.

"This has been a long time coming. And don't forget, you just gave me a Coke a while back. Let's use that hand truck."

Rat knew not to ask.

They duct-taped Hamner to the hand truck, and wheeled him out the door.

ONE-HUNDRED-ELEVEN

Ben scrambled into a cluttered storeroom. Simply breathing informed him it was adjacent to the boys' locker room.

Peter was launched toward his true identity, but Ben wasn't sure he had done enough to keep him on track. Johnson had to be the man who tried to capture Eve and shot Ray. Ben assumed Johnson was Will's boss, Frederick Moore. Now Ben had to save himself.

Groping in the dark, he found duffle bags full of baseballs, basketballs, and footballs—practice balls. He tripped over something he figured was a volleyball net. In one corner he found two ancient javelins with rusted metal tips. He put some baseballs in his knapsack, took the javelins, and folded the net over one shoulder.

If memory served, the locker room opened into a rear hall, and the gymnasium was a floor above. If he got to the front of the gym, the trophies and pictures in display cases would be to his right, and beyond them, the school's auditorium. He hoped to dash out the front entrance, bolt into the downtown areas, and make it back to his people.

Ben began to open the door very slowly. Someone yanked it open, poked a machine pistol into the room, and fired off a burst. Ben gave a horrific scream.

"Got him!" The shooter stepped into the doorframe. As he groped to one side and then the other for the light switch, searing pain pierced his abdomen. One flailing hand turned on a light. The last thing he saw was Ben Jordan rising from the floor, driving a javelin deeper and deeper through his gut.

Ben reached for the fallen man's weapon, but a burst of gunfire drove him back. Keeping low, he scuttled back out the door he'd first entered.

"That bastard killed George. He fucking speared him!"

"He speared him? Spread out. If you see him, if you think you know where he is, call for back up!"

Ben dug into his knapsack. He always carried certain unusual gear. From one small side pocket he fetched some fishing line and three lead sinkers, one slightly lighter that the others. He quickly tied precut lengths of stout braided line to each sinker and secured the line and sinker units to one another, and another line to where the units joined, creating a makeshift bolas. Thrown with reasonable precision, its cords could wind around and entangle a target's limbs. Even uninjured targets would find rapid escape or normal actions difficult.

Its silence was a plus. But the time and space to swing the bolas, step with the throw, and fling it cleanly counted against him. For precarious seconds, Ben could be a sitting duck.

Ben made his way to the ground floor and neared the exit doors. As he took a tentative first step toward the exit, an armed man stepped out of the gym to his right, and a voice to the left shouted, "There he is!"

Both men raised machine pistols. Neither could fire without putting his comrade at risk.

Dropping the second javelin Ben ran straight to his right, whirling the bolas. He kept between the men until he let loose at close range. Ben's bolas entangled the man's arms and entrapped his sub-machine gun. Ben cut behind him and dragged him along as a shield, ducking back into the gym. He pressed himself against the stacked bleachers and readied the net.

Both men followed. The first man rushed past Ben. The other followed, still struggling with the bolas, and noticed him.

"There he is!"

Ben threw the volleyball net over the first man and circled him twice, entrapping him and pulling him down. He stomped his neck hard, vaulted over him, and attacked the second.

Ben heard footsteps. He punched the second man's face with all his might and raced out of the gym, gunfire tearing up the floor behind him. Entering a stairwell once again, he climbed upstairs. Peering down the hall, he saw the back of an armed man walking away from him.

Ben put down his knapsack, and took out three hardballs. *That Johnson is sharp! It's been over twenty years since anyone connected me with the jock I used to be.* Ben got closer, wound up, beaned the man, and charged. The man staggered, turning in time for the second ball to strike him full in the face. Ben closed and drove his Bowie knife into the man's chest. Taking the man's weapon and clips, he dashed back down the stairwell to the basement.

Someone cried, "He's got to be in the stairwell. Two of you go to the second floor, two to the first, two get to the lower level. That should trap him. Let's finish this!"

If this was my op I'd pretend to pull out, and cover the escape routes I thought my target could take.

Then he heard, "New orders, boys! We have Gregorides and we've isolated Gilchrist. Forget this asshole for today. Move out."

And I'd be patient enough to make it convincing! Making for an exit would spring the trap. Checking the basement hallway, Ben saw men running toward both ends. He sprinted up rear stairs to the first floor, figuring where men would be stationed. Moving toward the front hall he risked a quick glance. A man was lying prone, facing away from him, with a perfect view of the doors in and out of the auditorium and gym, and the front entrance of the high school. Toward the other end of the hall, one door was slightly ajar. Probably the other man was there ready to back him if a target was identified.

Drawing closer to the prone marksman, Ben shoved the barrel of his gun against his spine and pricked his neck with the Bowie knife.

"That's my knife on your neck and my gun barrel on your spine. Your first sound is your last. Reach back. Take your cuffs. Cuff your right wrist. Bend your left leg back." Ben pulled the left cuff under the man's left thigh and clicked the other cuff on the man's left wrist behind him. He stuffed his handkerchief into the man's mouth.

"We're taking a trip." Ben pulled the man back down the main hall, and left him in a closet.

Ben popped through the gym, retrieving the second javelin. Exiting the rear of the gym, he traversed the long rear hall, and then the shorter side hall. He planned to circle behind the second man. The door of the principal's office remained ajar. The school secretary's office was between Ben and the principal's office. He slipped inside. A door between the two offices was open. An armed man with an H & K stood by the door to the hall, his back to Ben.

If I shoot him, everyone will know where I am. He's ten to twelve feet away. If he had to unholster, aim, and shoot a pistol, I'd have time. But he can just turn and fire. Yet with an eight foot javelin and two steps …

Ben positioned the javelin, took a deep breath, began to let it out … and then he charged, without a sound. The man collapsed.

Ben glanced into the hall. Nothing to be seen.

He pulled back. What to do next?

"Well, I think the party is over, Dr. Jordan. Throw your knapsack over to me. Eject the clip and anything you've chambered. Then throw the gun over here. At my feet."

Ben turned to see a tall, muscular blond man. He had a mild Swedish accent.

"Not from Stockholm?"

"Goteborg, for all the good it will do you. To the gym." He contacted his comrades. "Assemble at the gym."

As they walked, the Swede spoke. "Dr. Jordan. You are going to die. That is certain. But how you die remains under your control. Providing us with the information we require earns a quick shot to the head. Otherwise, someone you caused to be uncomfortable just a few days ago will gladly oversee your transition from this world to the next. Too bad time is so limited. I've never had the chance to see him at work, and I understand he is quite gifted. Trained by an old friend of yours."

"I have many old friends."

"Someone you spent a week with, long ago. A doctor who trains such people?"

"The world is full of brutal thugs."

"No! Dr. Kirchwasser is an artist, the best."

"Ah! The famous Dr. Kirchwasser! It's been so long. I don't even remember his first name."

"Anton. Herr Doctor Professor Anton Kirchwasser."

After all these years! Thanks to this cocky bastard, I finally know who tortured me! Flashbacks began to flood his mind, bringing up shards and fragments of horrific experiences long gone from memory. *After all these years! He's telling me because he's sure he'll watch me die. Herr Doctor Professor Anton Kirchwasser!*

They reached the gym. Four angry men awaited them.

"Merlin—he's yours. Stack weapons across the room, just in case." Ben was pushed down on the chair Johnson had used. *Soldiers, not cops! Again they didn't frisk me!*

Merlin turned to Ben, "Tell us all you know about Joe Morgan."

"Joe Morgan is the name given to Peter Souza by a group that recruits skilled covert operatives like yourselves and produces very specialized individuals by employing a range of behavioral techniques best summarized as brainwashing. He received aversive conditioning to disconnect him from his past and cause him to misperceive others' identities in a manner that might be used to make him hostile, even lethal, to those he loves and would normally protect.

"Joe Morgan was handled by someone who didn't pay any attention to his worsening headaches. He looked elsewhere for help. Instead of just taking care of his complaints, your people probably intensified his conditioning, and gave him instructions encouraging him to act out aggressively.

"So, he bolted. I was trying to bring him in for help and safety, and you guys have been trying to bring him in to keep your little party a private affair. I ran into him, told him you were a bunch of pricks, but I couldn't break through. He told me to get lost. I got another crack at him, right under your nose, but I didn't have enough time to mess up your programming."

"What else do you know?"

"Just what I told Johnson. If Will Rivers weren't an incompetent, narcissistic sadist, if he had Johnson's skill and moves, you'd just be loping along, just doing what you were doing."

"Anything more?"

"Yeah, Lars! Where's my consultation fee for identifying your internal organizational problems? You guys couldn't figure this out for yourselves."

Merlin pulled up Ben's shirt. He took a sheet of coarse sandpaper. "This will make you more open to the experience you imposed upon me."

"I hope you got extra points for getting back into the fight after that happened." Ben looked to the others. "Merlin really showed a lot of courage, Lars."

"Do you think that will get you anything, Jordan?"

Ben would be tortured with the capsaicin. Capsaicin inflicts a chemical burn. The damage done by a burn is not the result of the burn alone. That harm is augmented by a series of chemical processes, but some can be disrupted. Dabney Ewin, a New Orleans surgeon, discovered techniques by which hypnosis can trick the bodies of burn victims, shutting down some of those processes and minimizing damage. *Chemical burns have a lot in common with thermal burns. I've learned a lot from Dabney.*

By the time Merlin had scrubbed the rough sandpaper over Ben's abdomen and chest, leaving him raw and bleeding, Ben had already used his imagination to place himself in an ice-cold stream up to his neck, allowing the subjective experience of cold to dominate his body's responses. When Merlin poured capsaicin concentrate on his open wounds, somewhere in his mind Ben registered a mild discomfort—numb and cold.

Ben sat quietly, shivering but otherwise indifferent. Anticipating Merlin's next move, he imagined eating mint chocolate chip ice cream, and letting it slide down his throat until his mouth and throat became cold, painfully cold, and finally numb. In a corner of his mind he reminded himself, *Just like before, they didn't frisk me!*

Lars turned to Merlin. "What's going on here?"

"I'll get him!" Merlin opened another vial of the concentrate. "Hold his mouth open."

Lars forced Ben's mouth open. Merlin poured the vial's contents into Ben's mouth, and Lars held Ben's mouth shut.

"Now," Merlin predicted, "Now we'll see something!"

Ben sat quietly.

"Well, Dr. Jordan? What are you feeling?"

Ben shook his head, and uttered a low croak.

"Is he too badly burned to talk?" Lars asked.

"Maybe," said Merlin.

Ben uttered another croak.

"Whisper, Jordan!" Lars shook him.

Ben nodded. As Lars bent over to hear him, Ben spat a stream of capsaicin into his face. The big man stepped back and swung wildly, but Ben was already on his feet. He caught Merlin's head with both hands and smashed Merlin's face down on his knee. Still holding Merlin's head, he turned, pulling Merlin up behind him and sliding his hands down under Merlin's chin. As they momentarily stood back to back, Ben dipped a foot, wrenched Merlin's neck forward over his shoulder, and shot to his full height. Merlin's neck gave way with a sickening crack. Merlin's body fell to the floor, descending toward lifelessness, then deeper still.

For a moment the others stood stunned. When they ran for their weapons, Ben kicked the hindmost into the others. Leaping over them, he landed between them and their weapons. Lars staggered back to the fray.

Ben destroyed one man's knee, leaving him rolling in pain. For a moment two men grabbed Ben and held him while Lars landed an awesome punch. Ben felt one eye puffing up, his vision reduced to a slit.

Ben hooked a leg around the leg of one of those holding him. As Lars cranked up, Ben pulled the man toward him, pitching him between him and Lars. Kicking the falling man's spine, Ben pulled away from the second, and kicked at his head. That man blocked him, followed with a punch that threw Ben to the floor, and started to kick him.

Ben caught the stomping foot and twisted with all his strength. Something gave way. As the man collapsed, Ben's knife found his heart.

Before Ben recovered his knife, Lars caught him with another sledgehammer blow. His other eye began to close. Pushing aside Ben's weakened blocks, Lars wrapped him in a crushing bear hug.

"With my own hands, Ben Jordan! With my own hands!" Ben couldn't break free. His left arm was trapped against his chest. His right arm was pinned, useless, as if he were reaching for the sky. Lars had trapped Ben's right leg with his own. Ben's left foot dangled, barely touching the ground.

Ben fought off the pull of oblivion. Images flooded his mind—Yul Brynner in *The King and I. I'm dying and I see Yul Brynner? How fucked is that?* Ben struggled to pull air past the blockade of Lars's powerful grip. Other images floated through. A slender man stood before his karate class. His own teacher had arranged a demonstration by a visiting martial artist. Bald like Yul!

"Muay Thai is the art of eight limbs," said the visitor. "Elbows and knees join feet and fists." Ben lived to regret volunteering for a demonstration. The unfamiliar moves that left him bruised for months came back to him.

Ben willed himself to bring his right elbow down and his left knee up in unison. Lars tightened his grip even more.

Ben pumped his knee and struck down with his elbow. Nothing seemed to touch Lars until Ben had kneed and elbowed him over thirty times. Lars grunted and tried to tighten his hug. He could not make that happen.

Blood in the water! Ben fought with desperate fury. *Strike! Strike! Strike! Strike, or you'll never open your eyes again! Strike or Elani and the kids are lost forever! Strike or Eve and Peter and Maryellen lose their tomorrows! Strike or Kirchwasser wins, and escapes you for all eternity!*

"You're dying, Jordan," Lars taunted. "I'll send nice flowers. You'd have to hit me a hundred times before I'd even notice you were there!"

From somewhere inside Ben Jordan came a strange voice, strong and clear.

"I can do that!"

Ben picked up the pace of his attack. Lars felt himself weakening. He threw Ben to the ground hard and pounced. Ben rolled to the side and stunned Lars with an elbow to his head. Springing up, Ben put the weight of his entire body behind the single knee he smashed on Lars's neck. Lars lay still. He would lie still forever.

Retrieving his knife, Ben hobbled around to each fallen man. Those still alive he tied and hobbled with strips of cloth from their clothing. He collected their weapons, removed their clips and chambered rounds, and dragged them to the side of the bleachers. With one still-loaded machine pistol held in his lap he struggled to focus on the ice cream imagery, praying to quiet the fierce burning inside him.

ONE-HUNDRED-TWELVE

FBI, CIA, and NIS teams had arrived, with more on the way. Nicolai and Stover briefed them. Borodin was nowhere to be found. Ray's prisoners had been taken for processing. Hobbling toward the police station, he ran into Rat.

"Where's Jordan, Ray?" asked Rat.

"Let's find out."

"He said he'd look for Nick around the high school."

"Maybe he's still around there."

They borrowed a car and found the high school. They saw a body in the hall. Rat pulled out his .45. They passed the team pictures and trophies in the hall and looked into the gym. Its wooden floor was splintered by gunfire and littered with bodies and debris. Some bodies moved. Some did not.

They found Ben tucked into a corner behind a pile of guns. His face was swollen, his eyes reduced to narrow slits. He gave them a feeble wave and weak smile. He didn't try to rise. The Bowie knife and its sheath were at his side.

"You really don't play well with others," Ray commented.

"There should more outside the gym and on other floors."

"Are you gonna be big and bad like your asshole buddy Ray," Rat asked, "or can we get you some help?"

"I think they kicked the big and bad out of me, 'specially that big guy Lars. Don't move me, either."

"Neck?"

"Might be. Let's play it safe. I'm full of that pepper extract. Get me a few gallons of ice cream, milk, and peanut butter. Mint chocolate chip, or anything."

"Ray, you're the doc," said Rat. "Stay with this underachiever and I'll get a Boy Scout or someone else who knows first aid." He slid Ben's Bowie knife into its sheath. "The way you make friends, you'll need your toy."

"There are still a few of them out there, guys."

"Probably fewer than you think, Ben."

"Ray, I need a favor from you. Tell this to Lucco, too. I may have a concussion. I could forget something really important. Remember the name Dr. Anton Kirschwasser for me."

"Sure. Because?"

"I owe him something. Oh! Send big Lars nice flowers."

Ray stood by until the EMTs took Ben out on a stretcher.

ONE-HUNDRED-THIRTEEN

Lurking behind a building near the police station and parking lot, Johnson glanced toward the street. A staging area had been set up in a parking lot in front of the police station. One ambulance pulled away. An injured man was loaded on to the other. One stretcher remained behind. The man on this stretcher, propped up on an elbow, wore a neck collar and licked an ice-cream cone. A young EMT spoke to him briefly. The man nodded, waved him off, and kept after that ice cream. The EMT left with the second ambulance.

One of Johnson's backup vehicles was parked barely 200 feet away. Reach it, and he could be on a Program boat within minutes. Reluctantly, he acknowledged the wisdom of the saying, "He who fights and runs away will live to fight another day." *And payback will be a bitch!* His superiors would help him cover his trail after he did his part, destroying anyone who might compromise him or Glenville-Rogers. Will Rivers, Marty Franks, the Nicks, and their handlers would be sacrificed. Put in place by parties far above Johnson, Lou would be exempt. Those further down would be left disconnected from the upper levels of their former command. Their fates were of no interest to the Program, but to avoid the unlikely possibility of backlash, International Logistics would go bankrupt. Everyone would receive generous severance packages, and life would go on.

Nearing the front of the building, Johnson saw people milling around, people on the ground, people in handcuffs or plastic cuff ties under the watchful eyes of guards, and people standing in small groups talking animatedly with one another. He recognized Eve Gilchrist with some tall young man, Stover and his son, the Souza family, and others. Annibal Cabral, flanked by his sons, was receiving treatment for his abrasions from EMTs. Body bags offered grim testimony that some, probably his own men, had passed beyond help.

Johnson's Heckler & Koch MP5SD with its cut down stock and suppressor lay ready in his unzipped gym bag. A hammerless aluminum .38 Smith & Wesson Model 42 rested in his ankle holster.

Johnson averted his face from the man on the stretcher. One of his own might recognize him, cry for help, and ruin him. Glenville-Rodgers's strategists and lawyers would decide whether those captured would be liberated, bribed, or taken out no matter where they were.

Leaving the stretcher behind him, his car was mere seconds away. He heard a soft clunk and dragging sound at his feet. Looking down, he watched a bass plug with large treble hooks leap up, catch the leg of his khakis, and bite into his flesh.

"It's Johnson! It's Johnson! Get him! Get him!"

The man on the stretcher, the man with the neck collar and a swollen face from hell, had hooked him and was screaming for help. Their eyes locked.

"Jordan!"

Ben struggled to stay on his feet, working the stubby collapsible rod. He jerked its tip upward. The hooks bit deeper and Johnson was pulled off balance.

He went down and Ben tried to keep him down, dragging him from side to side. The rod snapped. Ben stumbled. Johnson caught the line and trapped it under one foot. Wrapping it around his hand, he yanked sharply with every ounce of his desperate strength. Already off balance when the line gave way, Ben fell. Johnson snapped off two rounds from the .38. One grazed Ben's head. He collapsed.

The crowd stared at Johnson. Pacella and Tomaselli charged, revolvers already drawn, and Prentice James sped past them. Lucco, the salami man, produced a .45 magnum, screaming Italian obscenities as he ran. Chief Dowling dashed toward his own car. He'd have a shotgun, maybe worse. A man with the build of a retired linebacker and a wiry bearded biker were charging hard—they'd all be on him in moments.

Johnson dropped to one knee, freed up his Heckler & Koch, and fired a burst over the heads of the crowd.

"Back off, and no one gets hurt" he shouted. Some quickly hit the ground. But most stood frozen like deer transfixed by headlights. Johnson wanted to finish Ben Jordan, but he couldn't risk turning his back on this crowd. Not for a second!

Change of plans! Leaning against the building's weathered wood, he aimed directly at the crowd.

"You two and the other cops, toss your weapons on the ground. You too, big guy! Everybody come up close. I'll tell you when to stop. Otherwise I just start shooting."

He kept the machine pistol pointed toward Eve, Mrs. Souza, and Sarah Fletcher, all standing together. The crowd drew near. Buchholz moved to Eve's side. Lucco Brazzo and Rat bided their time, waiting for an edge, waiting for an opening.

"Everybody get real close together. There's no place to hide. Chief, here's what's going to happen! I'm getting out of here. You're driving me. You'd be a great hostage, Congressman Stover, but I know you were a SEAL. Dr. Gilchrist! You get in front with the sheriff. That little girl! What's your name?"

"Sarah."

"Sarah sits in the back with me."

"No! No!" Jill cried.

Mrs. Souza fell to her knees, raising her hands as if in prayer. "Please! Leave the child alone."

Jim Cabot started to come out of the crowd, "Leave her alone. Take me."

Johnson fired a shot near his feet. "Not today, hero!"

"Dowling! Strip to your underwear and bring that cruiser around. If you even look like you're thinking of something I don't like, the ladies get it first."

Johnson scanned the crowd and gestured toward Mrs. Souza.

"You want to help this little girl? You're going to be my shield until Dowling brings the cruiser around."

There was a murmur in the crowd.

"Everyone quiet. What did someone say?"

Mr. Souza spoke softly. "A lot of us are scared. A lot of us are Portuguese. A couple of us were saying *The Lord's Prayer* in Portuguese."

"Pray all you want, but not out loud. Get up here, lady!"

"Please, sir," Mr. Souza spoke. "My wife is terrified."

Johnson pointed his machine pistol directly at Mrs. Souza.

"All right! All right! Let me say it in Portuguese."

Mr. Souza whispered comfortingly as he supported his terrified wife. Finally, she nodded and began to walk toward Johnson, trembling and weeping, unable to raise her head and look at the face of the man who tried to enslave her son. The closer she drew, the more Mrs. Souza faltered. Her legs seemed ready to buckle at any moment.

Less than five feet from Johnson, she collapsed to the ground.

"Get up! Now!"

Mrs. Souza raised her head and locked her eyes on Johnson. She raised her hands slowly, imploringly. Her left hand stayed low. It was empty. Her clenched right hand shot forward, hurling a cloud of loose dirt into Johnson's face. His hands went to his eyes. "I'll kill you, bitch!" Wiping his eyes and trying to regain control, Johnson never saw Mrs. Souza flatten herself on the ground.

ONE-HUNDRED-FOURTEEN

It was hard to hear the low hiss, the soft whoosh, even in the still summer air. For a fraction of a second, three feet of iron mounted on six feet of dark, stout oak flashed in the sun. It was easier to hear the soft dull thud and startled grunt that followed.

Frederick Moore, Mike Johnson, whoever he was, grunted again and started to collapse. But his body refused to fall. He tried to make sense of the shaft of polished wood on the metal object protruding from his chest. He wondered why his hands lost their grips on his Heckler & Koch and his .38. His mind clouded over before he heard the sounds of his weapons hitting the ground, before he could fathom that his body was transfixed by a nineteenth-century whaler's harpoon, pinned to the wooden building behind him like a butterfly in a museum showcase. Another soft thud—the harpoon's oaken shaft detached and fell to the ground. His eyes glazed, closed, and saw no more.

Philippe Sousa, eighty-six years of age, stood as erect and strong as the day he lowered away as harpooner in the prow of Boat 2. A grim smile briefly crossed his weathered face. Then he turned, and walked away without saying a word.

ONE-HUNDRED-FIFTEEN

Chief Dowling was a wily man. He had devised an ingenious series of prison annexes. In addition to boat holds and stores, over a dozen very waterlogged men in handcuffs or plastic wrist ties had been accommodated near the deep end of a pool at The White Elephant Hotel. They were encouraged to remain in a state of marination by the patchwork coalition of locals recruited and mobilized by Prentice James. Restaurant workers with fiendish grins and nasty butcher's knives circled the pool. Prentice had passed the word to a current Whaler fullback, who abdicated his summer job and called other teammates. Another ring formed, consisting of current and past players from the high school's football team and the outraged parents of Nantucket Whalers past and present. Some of Nicolai's frat brothers, searching for an early drink, went looking for Noah, and were drawn by the commotion. Josie, too savvy and too nosy to be fooled, had called a tree surgeon she knew. Things long and sharp were brought to poolside, and wielded with enthusiasm. Johnson's men soaked in the harsh sun, under the "make my day" scrutiny of all assembled.

A handful of men had brought shotguns or deer rifles, and kept them aimed directly at their captives' heads. The tree surgeon brought along a chainsaw. He was pleased to power it up from time to time, providing a further incentive for Johnson's men to remain drenched and demure.

Back at the hospital several surgeons continued to work on the man who crossed Ambassador Gilchrist. Despite two transfusions and over 350 sutures, much remained to be done.

Johnson and the man skewered by Jim's penny nails were encased in thick body bags. Other body bags were carried from the high school; several other men were carried out on stretchers.

Seated in a collapsible wheelchair, his neck in a brace and his head swathed in blood-soaked bandages, Ben kept forcing down the ice cream. Ray sat in another, his wounds no longer oozing.

Rat brought them cold drinks, muttering, "I always knew psychiatrists were fucking crazy!"

Toward evening a pair of CIA agents patrolling Nantucket Harbor noticed something very much out of the ordinary. Suspended fifteen feet above them from the mast of a large sailboat, a hand truck swung on a stout line. It contained a man who once had owned a pearl-handled revolver and a stolen medicine bag with a silver and turquoise clasp. He turned slowly in the breeze.

ONE-HUNDRED-SIXTEEN

Thanks to the efforts of Mark, Rat, Admiral Marshall, and the Coast Guard, reinforcements were on the scene. Helicopters had brought in NIS, FBI, and CIA contingents. Prisoners were being processed rapidly and transported out by the same helicopters to secure military and federal prisons. The jail was seriously overcrowded as the men from the annex jails were transported to the central location.

When Ray hobbled into the station, Chief Dowling waved a greeting. "The phones are working again. The men I sent by ferry? The ferry crews found them tied and unconscious in men's room stalls, without their IDs. Those bastards were tough."

"May I?" asked Ray. "There was a call Ben wanted me to make."

"Go ahead."

Ray put a call in to Louie. Amazingly, he reached him.

"I hadda come in for a leaky toilet. What?"

"I'm calling for Dr. Jordan, the man who fought those guys at your place. He's assisting the police. We understand that you got a good look at one of the men who tried to kidnap Dr. Gilchrist. Can you describe him?"

"Gotta to finish up with the toilet. Give me a couple minutes."

As Ray awaited the callback, a handsome young man presented his credentials to the chief.

"Patrick Flynn, CIA. I'm with a team that will be taking these people out in small groups. Other teams are doing the same. I hope they know about us, but we all seem to be flying by the seat of our pants today."

"Well, Flynn, the way things have been, I double-check everything."

Ray got his callback. While he listened and took notes, he watched the two prisoners just front of him, freshly plucked from the pool. Their glances back and forth and their intense interest in Flynn made him curious.

"Thanks for getting back to me."

"Yeah. You want a description of the guy who screwed me over?"

"Please."

Louie began to describe the man he knew as Junior. Ray tried not to react. The description applied very well to someone close at hand.

"I need your help for just a few minutes more, sir." He had noticed a discolored purple fingernail on the index finger of Flynn's right hand. "Any distinguishing marks?"

"Yeah. Looks like he hit his finger with a hammer. Index finger. Don't ask me which one. Well, maybe the right."

"Anything else you want to tell me?" asked Ray.

"Sure. Hey, that bastard Junior made me look bad. I want a piece of him."

"Sounds like a plan. Hold on." Ray addressed the new arrival. "Excuse me, Agent Flynn, this is about a lost dog. Routine stuff doesn't come to a halt just because everything is hitting the fan. This one is a pit bull. It's scaring people." He passed a note to the chief.

Dowling scanned it and nodded.

"Bear with me," Ray pretended to place the call from Louie on hold, and said into the phone. "Oh? Damn well about time," Ray smiled. "Hey, Agent Flynn. I've got a guy on the phone who can give us a description of another one of them. I'm just a civilian. This sounds important. Let me put you on the phone with this valuable eye-witness."

Ray said to Louie, "Sir, I'm putting you on the line with a real CIA agent. Describe that bastard to him."

Ray stood up as he handed Flynn the phone. Louie made him.

In moments "Agent Flynn" was whispering "Louie!" and Louie was screaming, "Junior, you fucking bastard!" loudly enough for Ray and Dowling to hear. Junior went for his gun, but Dowling smashed him in the face. Junior crashed to the floor, spitting teeth and gushing blood. Ray went to the floor. Junior tried to shake his head clear and reach for his leg holster, but Ray's elbow smashed the top of Junior's skull. His body went into a prolonged, grotesque seizure.

The two men in the chairs swore and cursed. Ray could hear Louie shouting, "What the hell is going on? Will someone tell me what the hell is going on?"

The phone had fallen to the floor. Ray crawled over.

"Hey, Louie? You there, man?"

"Yeah. What happened?"

"Was it OK with you that the chief and I just hit Junior in the head a couple times? That his face is all busted up? That his teeth are all over the floor? When you ID'd him he freaked and we had to knock him down. How many teeth? Well, at least three that I can see right near him. Loser? No. Not you. If you didn't ID him, I'd be a dead man and he might have pulled off a jailbreak. In my book, you're a hero!"

Dowling took the phone. "Hey, Louie? I hope you can handle getting a medal? You can? Good."

ONE-HUNDRED-SEVENTEEN

Betty Gilchrist had monitored Coast Guard transmissions once the new radio was installed. She came from a yachting family. Among the Gilchrists, Betty was acknowledged to be the best sailor.

She had obeyed her husband's orders to stay hidden. Three cars drove into the marina's lot. A number of men, some clearly armed, clambered aboard a large powerboat docked nearby.

Betty radioed Admiral Marshall. His wife answered. They went to another channel and Admiral Marshall took the microphone.

"Please make message as before and say approximately one dozen armed men boarding vessels, preparing for departure."

"Keep out of this. I'll call the Coast Guard. Stand by."

In moments the Admiral called back. "All Coast Guard resources continue deployed in marine rescue situations. Just lay low."

"No can do. Contact the police or whatever. The wind is coming up. Tell them I can give them twenty minutes to arrive on site. Over and out."

Betty slowly unfurled half of her boat's dark colored jib. She tied a slender line to her stout forward mooring line, and fastened its other end to a fender line amidships. She released the forward line itself and let it sink. The breeze swung her bow out, slowly crossing the channel between the docks and bay. With equally adept seamanship, Betty screamed,

"Oh, my God! What's happened to my line! Sam! Sam! Where is that man! Sam! Did you sneak off with that awful blonde tramp on that Catalina 30? You did! You did!"

And Betty began to wail. As she wailed louder and louder, *Cricket's Caper* continued to drift. With every passing moment its bow blocked more and more of the passageway vessels relied upon to reach the marina from the bay, or depart the marina for the bay beyond.

ONE-HUNDRED-EIGHTEEN

The admiral contacted Dowling. Cabral, Stover, Rat, and Nicolai were at the station.

"Amazing lady! What can we do?"

Stover and Cabral nodded as one. Stover took command.

"On presidential authority I'm commandeering all 'copters here and incoming. Load 'em with shooters." He pointed to a map. "Land fire teams at these locations. I go with the first, Annibal with the second, Nicolai with the third."

"Too busted up to lead, Stove, but I'll go with you," said Cabral. "Let NIS go with us—all Navy. Let Nicolai honcho the Company boys in their special 'copter. Rat was recon. He rescued Mark. Put Rat, the Philly three, and some FeeBees in the third, and get out of their way."

ONE-HUNDRED-NINETEEN

Betty Gilchrist, fluttery and hysterical, epitomized helplessness.

Men screamed at her. She dissolved in tears.

"I know! I know!" she sobbed, "My husband won't show me how to do anything. He's afraid I'll break something or run into somebody. Please don't yell at me! Could you find it in your hearts to bring my boat back to the dock? I'm such a fool!"

"We gotta help her," one man said. "No choice!"

Men came on board with a new line. Betty prepared ice tea and offered them cookies. The men mumbled their thanks and tried to start the engine. But Betty had anticipated they would try to use it to bring *Cricket's Caper* back to dockside. The fuel line was clamped at a very obscure location.

The men encountered difficulty pulling the bow back to dockside with manpower alone. They didn't notice the partially unfurled jib that made their work much more difficult.

Hearing the faint sounds of a helicopter in flight, Betty came around with ice tea again. "That looks so hard. Are you sure you don't want to take a break?"

Finally, one man noticed the jib. The sail furled and secured, the others went ashore to secure a forward line. The sound of helicopters grew louder.

"Secure the bow! Get under way. I'll jump on when you come alongside."

A helicopter descended over the marina's parking lot. Elias Stover's voice came over a bullhorn.

"Attention men at dockside and on board dockside vessels. Raise your hands. You are about to be taken into custody under the joint authority of federal, military, and local law enforcement agencies. If you resist arrest, we will open fire!"

The men bolted toward their own boat. The man on *Cricket's Caper* shouted, "Don't panic! That's no gunship. We can knock them out of the sky. We'll take this woman hostage. They won't stop us!"

An unmarked black helicopter came in from the bay. Nicolai announced,

"Attention men at dockside and on board *Cricket's Caper*. You were correct. The first helicopter was not a gunship. This one is."

"They've got nothing!" shouted the man on *Cricket's Caper*, standing on the bow, "Ahoy! We are holding this woman hostage!" He turned to point to Betty Gilchrist, who knocked him overboard with a boat hook.

Now a third helicopter hovered off the motor craft's beam. There was muffled noise, then an unexpected explosion.

"I am Lieutenant Pacella of the Philadelphia PD. You are cowardly shits. You fuck over the young and innocent. You make war on women and children. Please give me an excuse to send you from this world to the next. I'm begging you! Please!"

"He's crazy," a man shouted.

Stover thought of Mark.

"He's talking for every one of us," he bellowed.

Now Rat spoke. "Sounds like a plan. The men and women of the Coast Guard you've screwed with all day send greetings. Two armed cutters are minutes away. They respectfully request that you give them good cause to send your sorry asses to hell."

* * *

A few minutes later Betty Gilchrist removed the clamp from her fuel line and radioed her thanks to Admiral Marshall, who was overcome with emotion. His wife spoke for him, "The admiral doesn't quite know what to say when the hero is a woman. But he's a quick learner. Brava, Betty! Brava!"

ONE-HUNDRED-TWENTY

The Philly three were saying their goodbyes. The Stovers and Cabrals had already left to begin repairs on *Os Lusiadas*. The Souzas were at home, overwhelmed and exhausted. Grandfather Philippe had opened a bottle of *vino verde*, enjoyed a single glass, and went to sleep. Peter had called Maryellen. They would meet for coffee the next morning. He and Sean Fletcher were upstairs renewing their friendship. Bobby Gray finally convinced Ray to have his wounds redressed and crash in a nearby hotel. Rat brought in dinner for the threesome from The Scrimshaw Duck. Prentice James and Chief Dowling, along with others, were putting the station back in order.

"Time for us to go," said Lucco. "We gotta get an early start tomorrow. Only ferry we could get was so f … so very early." They shook hands all around. Then Lucco turned to Ambassador and Betty Gilchrist. "Your wife and your daughter are truly amazing. And you, sir, you scare me."

Eve rose and kissed all three men. Then she gave a second kiss to Lucco. "You'll always be very special to me," she said.

Lucco took her hand and placed it in Jim's. "My Mama told me to do that. And she said that you better take damn good care of the Cricket or she'll send the wrath of God after you."

"You mean you'll come after me?" asked Jim.

"No," said Tomaselli. "His Mama will come after you. That's much worse."

Borodin knocked. "There's someone who wants to thank you on behalf of the nation. I don't have much time to set up the connection. Another guy is working outside. Can I get some help with the cameras? My friend here looks exhausted."

Indeed, Nicolai sat snoring in a corner. Several men lent a hand. Coach Mack's living room quickly filled with lights and boxes. From the boxes, Borodin removed two cameras and mounted them on tripods.

"One will cover the couch and these chairs for a group shot. I'll man the other for individual and close-up shots."

He looked at his watch.

"I should contact the technical people on the other end. Right back." A voice came through Borodin's headphones.

Eve looked around. She seemed distressed.

"Where's my Dad?"

Ambassador Gilchrist came into the room moments later.

"Mom's still freshening up. She'll be right down." He looked around. "Wow! What's all the excitement about? Are you upset, Cricket?"

"Well, Dad, it seems like we're getting a call from Washington. And, I don't know. There's something about the guy who's setting it up. Or maybe it's the voice coming through the earphones. Something is giving me the creeps."

There were sounds outside.

"Just me with some extra cables," shouted Borodin. More sounds came from behind the house.

Ambassador Gilchrist shrugged, "Well, Cricket … Wait a minute! The president … He should be at on his way to Belgium by now."

"Too late, Mr. Ambassador," came the voice from outside. "Sorry, folks. Gotta do what I gotta do."

"That's the voice. It came through the earphones. He said the same words before they tortured me. 'Gotta do what I gotta do.' I recognize that voice."

"Right you are, Dr. Gilchrist! Don't even try to leave. The windows and doors are rigged to blow."

Lucco Brazzo checked.

"Yeah. Everything's rigged. But I figure if we ram the door with that long couch, we could blow it and make a break for it."

"My guess is that he ..." Ben stopped to tear open what appeared to be a box of cables. "Oh, no!" It was packed with explosives. He found more in the other equipment boxes. "Wake up Nicolai!"

Buchholz shook Nicolai awake.

He staggered over.

"What the hell?"

Nicolai collapsed as he tried to focus on the bomb.

"Sorry. My vision is so blurry. I must have been drugged. Tell me what you see!"

Pacella drew in close. He attempted to describe the set-up while Tomaselli and Brazzo tried to see what the two men were doing.

"It looks like they're still messing with some wires," said Tomaselli.

"To two boxes," Brazzo added.

"That's a clunky set-up. We must have knocked out their first team," said Nicolai.

"What's the roof like near where he's working?" Ben asked.

"Steep angle under our son's attic room," said Mack. "He's still up there with Pete."

"What does that room overlook?"

"A roof over the front porch. A whole floor down. My boy used to sneak ..."

Ben tried to sprint up the stairs, but the best he could manage were clumsy lurches, tripping as he went. Upstairs, the boys had been talking. Peter fiddled with a tacky letter opener with a fake scrimshaw handle. "Greetings from Nantucket!" was stamped in red on one side.

"What are you doing with this piece of crap?"

"Oh, that? I was going to send it to this cheerleader I met when we played Somerset, but she shot me down before I ever mailed it." Clutching a fist to his "broken heart," Sean fell to the floor. "Shot down again!" They were still laughing when Ben struggled into Sean's room.

"What's going on, Dr. Jordan?"

"That bastard outside is fixing to blow the house …"

Nick beat him to the window.

"The other guy is my roommate, Marty Franks! Shit! He was a fake, too!"

Only the first floor had been wired. The boys opened the window noiselessly. Sean pulled a rope ladder from under his bed and slipped it over the sill. Before Ben could move, Peter Souza waved him back and slipped out without a sound.

Once on the porch roof, Peter Souza silently rose to his full height, stretched, and then sunk into a sprinter's crouch.

Ben whispered to Sean, "Go into the next bedroom over and make noise, but stay low."

Ben tapped Peter with the ladder to get his attention. Ben made the football sign for "time out." Then he held up two fingers, folded one, and then the second. The noise began. Borodin and Franks looked toward the noise.

Peter sprang forward, took three powerful strides, and threw himself, head first, at Borodin. Borodin had just squeezed off a shot and heard Sean scream when Peter tackled him and took him down hard. Borodin's gun clattered down the pavement, skidding under the pick-up truck that had carried the explosives. Borodin sprang up and shoved Peter away. Peter charged

Borodin, but Borodin drove him back again and dropped him to the ground with a fusillade of vicious kicks. Leaving Peter stunned and breathless, Borodin returned to Franks and the boxes.

Ben was too battered to make a jump. He was afraid he might set off explosives if he stumbled or fell. Sean felt his way into the room, blood flowing down over his face from a scalp wound.

"I'm OK. It just needs pressure."

Peter sprang to the attack once more, braving terrible kicks from Borodin while trying to fend off Peter Franks as well. When Franks grappled with Peter, Borodin made for two containers alongside the pick-up truck. Atop each container was a small dark box, both flashing a series of blinking lights.

Peter screamed, "It's radio-controlled! Shoot out the transmitters! Shoot out both!" Borodin took over. He threw Peter down and tried to pound his head against the ground. No one noticed the noiseless exits of Lucco Brazzo and Ambassador Gilchrist.

"He's going to kill him!" Eve screamed.

Heavy footsteps thundered down the roof. Lucco Brazzo landed badly, and cursed in pain.

"The fat fucker broke his leg!" Borodin crowed, and went after Peter again. Again, Peter was thrown to the ground. Borodin ran toward him. Suddenly Borodin disappeared.

"Fat fucker! This fat fucker is kicking your ass!" Broken leg and all, Lucco crawled back and brought Borodin to the ground. He pounded Borodin with all his might.

"That's as far as I can go, Pete. You got the ball."

Borodin would be dead long before Lucco stopped punching.

Inside the house, a calm, refined voice, gone cold as ice, spoke softly as two bullets the size of cigars were inserted into the chambers of a double rifle.

"Get away from the window," Ambassador Gilchrist ordered. He cradled a Purdey .470 Nitro gently in his arms, like a big game hunter on safari. Betty Gilchrist stood behind him, her arm resting gently on her husband's shoulder.

"Ray, I hear you acquired a knife today, Ray. Use it."

Ray cut through the top and right side of a screen window and pulled back the freed corner, opening a triangular space.

"Much obliged."

In a smooth unhurried motion, Ambassador Gilchrist brought the massive weapon to bear and destroyed the first transmitter. Fragments of metal and plastic showered down on Peter Souza and Marty Franks. Peter went on the attack. Neither man was trying to win. Each was trying to kill the other. Their struggle blocked the second transmitter from view.

Franks faked out Peter with a series of high jabs, and then kicked below Peter's defense, landing a vicious kick to his crotch. As Peter collapsed Franks lurched toward the second transmitter, pulled it from its protective casing and carried it to the bed of his pick-up, blocked from sight. Peter struggled to his feet but would never reach Marty in time.

Marty hit a remote detonator switch and turned his full fury against Peter. *So that old fart brought in his museum piece for show and tell, and got in a lucky shot. No way that happens again!*

"Stay away from the window," said the ambassador. "Stay away."

"How's this going to go, sir?" asked Buck. Without a word, Betty Gilchrist squeezed her husband's arm, and stood back.

"I wanted this old Purdey to complete the big five." Again, the smooth, practiced motion as Ambassador Gilchrist brought the .470 Nitro to bear.

Buchholz saw canisters on the pick-up's bed. What was Gilchrist thinking? The .470 discharged. Its heavy slug, designed to drop charging African elephants and Cape buffalos in their tracks, pierced every canister. Fluid splattered in every direction. But the transmitter?

Franks screamed in triumph.

"You're gone, you pathetic losers! Gone!" He sprinted away from the inevitable blast.

Nothing happened.

Franks raced back to the truck. What was wrong? Everything was wet! He reached into the truck bed and his hand came back wet. Outside of its case, the transmitter was vulnerable to any liquid—even to the water from the canisters Borodin and Franks had used to shield their equipment from view! Its lights flickered no more. It had drowned.

A powerful forearm compressed Marty Franks's throat. What was that mounting pressure in his back? What was that sharp discomfort building into excruciating pain, into agony piercing deeper and deeper into his body? Why did something seem to twist as it made its way further and further into his core? Why did his lower back feel so wet?

"One good stab in the back deserves another, Marty."

Peter Souza controlled Marty Franks's slumping body as it slid to the ground. Then he knelt with him, never releasing his chokehold until the job was done. By the pale light from the Fletchers' windows, Peter still could see a white handle protruding from Borodin's back. Sean's long-unsent gift had finally arrived at a meaningful address. "Greetings from Nantucket!" said Peter Henry Souza. "Greetings from Nantucket!"

"Amen to that, my brother," said Lucco Brazzo.

ONE HUNDRED-TWENTY-ONE

At FBI headquarters in Washington, DC, Associate Director Lawrence Middleton dictated a report:

"Medical personnel at Nantucket Cottage Hospital contacted this office on behalf of Agent Howard Dunlop. Agent Dunlop went missing en route to Nantucket to provide assistance and support to Congressman Stover. He was attacked aboard a ferry bound for Nantucket and found a day later unconscious, bound, and gagged, in a maintenance locker aboard that ferry. He had suffered head trauma. His identification stolen, he was hospitalized as a John Doe. Upon regaining consciousness, Dunlop insisted his report be transmitted ASAP. His assailant's description matches that of a man who died subsequent to injuries suffered while attempting to free prisoners from police custody in Nantucket."

ONE HUNDRED-TWENTY-TWO

Elani's voice was bright and happy. "I've had a wonderful time with Rakel and Danielle. I'll visit the kids on my way back. How have things been the last few days? I haven't been able to reach you."

"I was swamped for a while, but things are quieter now."

"Are you keeping busy enough with that mind control case?"

"It's just been creeping along. One part of it is resolving well. The rest may take a long time. Anyhow, it's a slow day in Gladwyne. I can't wait to see you."

"Ben, you keep telling me it's a slow day in Gladwyne. But it's never a slow day wherever you are. You're not in Gladwyne, are you?"

ONE HUNDRED-TWENTY-THREE

A few months later, at the academic year's first grand rounds in psychiatry, Ray Hawkes and Ben Jordan listened proudly as Bobby Gray introduced Jeffrey Kane, who in turn gave an effusive but scholarly introduction to Homer Spence, an internationally celebrated expert who had not given a public lecture in many years. Changes in the grand rounds schedule were announced. A special lecture would be given by Ray Hawkes, whose book would be published the following spring. This would replace a previously announced talk by Will Rivers, who had suddenly taken a sabbatical year at an undisclosed location.

* * *

Eve Gilchrist and Jim Cabot were en route to visit Eve's parents overseas. Elani, a skilled jeweler, had repaired Eve's broken necklace as good as new. But for this trip, Eve had left wearing a new piece of jewelry as well, an elegant but smaller piece of jewelry with a single brilliant stone that made her very, very happy.

* * *

Ambassador and Betty Gilchrist sat together in a very private room. Short of an international crisis or an imminent attack on the embassy by terrorist hordes, no one dared to disturb them in the ambassador's modest workroom, a far cry from his formal and elegant ceremonial office, where most embassy visitors assumed he performed his duties. Two comfortable armchairs and a daily sweep for bugs made this unremarkable room a perfect sanctuary, where they could talk without fear of being overheard.

The Gilchrists were fond enough of their future son-in-law, this highly eligible Boston Brahmin radiologist, but since Eve would be the first of their children to marry, they were entering new and unfamiliar territory. As they shared a gentle kiss, toasting one another with green ice tea, their eyes drifted to a picture taken just before Marty Franks's final plan went into action. Everyone looked tired and disheveled, except Eve, who somehow carried off looking pert and fresh in any situation. The ambassador's eyes wandered to the left of that picture, where a shattered electronic device was mounted on a fine walnut panel. To the right of the picture, nailed directly to another walnut panel, a large water canister was on display. It bore the conspicuous impact of a large caliber bullet.

"Well, my dear," said the ambassador's wife. "Now those are really impressive trophies!"

"I was tempted to mount the grill of that pick-up, but I really only wounded the beast after dealing with that big jug and its evil comrades. It wouldn't have been sporting."

"I must admit, I'm not quite sure whether or not you're serious."

"I'm a diplomat, dear. You're not supposed to be sure."

* * *

Prentice James had begun training in a police academy out of town. Nantucket had no academy of its own. His instructors considered him outstanding. They urged him to make his career in the city where he was being trained. However, his return to Chief Dowling's department in Nantucket was eagerly awaited by many, but by no one more than Prentice James.

* * *

Maria Nunez's new chair wrote to her former chief at MGH, "It's enough to make me wonder whether sometimes a great force intervenes and directs things. Our patients are convinced Dr. Nunez is an angel of mercy. They've never met anyone who takes so much time and makes such an effort to understand them and their problems."

* * *

Lucco Brazzo made a full recovery. Jim Cabot made a special trip to Philadelphia to ask him to be one of his groomsmen when he married Eve. The couple made Mama and Papa promise to attend as their honored guests. Tony Pacella's daughter was accepted to medical school at the U, and Frank Tomaselli became grandfather of twins. Hard to recognize without his sneer, he walked around in a state of uncharacteristic and inexpressible joy, with an infinitely expanding number of photographs to show. Daniel Cabral was enjoying every blood- and sweat-stained day of the demanding training that brought him closer to becoming a SEAL. Christophe was in his glory as a feared linebacker and lady-killer at New Bedford High. Assistant coaches and wealthy alumni from major football powers were scouting him every week.

The teams of Coaches Buchholz and Fletcher were off to good starts, but had yet to face New Bedford. Mark Stover became an Eagle Scout. Ben, Tomasso, Annibal, Rat, Chief Dowling, and Admiral Marshall attended the Stover family's celebration.

* * *

Peter Souza declined treatment for the moment. He decided to spend a year with his family, reestablishing his roots. He went fishing with his grandfather every day. Peter and Maryellen shyly renewed their long-interrupted relationship. Peter talked a lot with Coach Mack about becoming a teacher.

Maryellen Madeiros began to take courses at Cape Cod Community College. She knows she is good enough.

* * *

Ray would be forever silent about how his interview techniques extracted precise information disclosing Johnson's sleepers and their handlers. He remained inordinately modest about his accomplishment and uncomfortable with the praise he received. All too often Ray had endured unjustified derision and scorn. He slowly learned to endure unjustified praise. No masked man appeared in any account or report. In the depths of his being, Ray understood that a sudden twist in the tangled skein of a complex life had provided a bereaved son a way to express his profound love for the MIA father he could barely remember. The masked man who did not exist, keeping faith with the father who survived only in the shadowy realm of his childhood memories, reached out to bring these MIAs hidden in plain sight back to their homes and those who kept their memories alive. Now at least no man named Nick would be left behind. Other hidden victims could and would be found. Other actions could and would be taken.

* * *

A year later, along a winding rural road on the western slopes of Pennsylvania's Allegheny Mountains, the roar of six monster choppers shattered the pastoral calm. Six men rode in formation, two by two. Spider and Rat were followed by Cracker and Crusty. Behind them rode two others, one rather young, one middle-aged, both still almost clean-shaven, slowly working their ways into their undercover identities. Alert, attentive, and smiling, they immersed themselves in the moment and drank deeply of a new and unexpected intoxication. They rejoiced in the strangely erotic embrace of the wind that rushed to kiss their faces with the ardor of an eager lover. They succumbed to the alluring touch of breezes that caressed their bodies as they streamed on past, at once relaxing and exciting with their gentle urgency. Modeling the skills of the more experienced bikers, they leaned into the curves and swerves, and their bodies responded to the engrossing sensual harmonies that resonated between their machines and the roads that traversed the ever-changing terrain. They were seduced.

As they swung around a long gentle curve, Rat looked back at his new companions, smiled, and raised his fist in a salute. Nicolai Rimsky-Korsakoff and Frank Tomaselli grinned back like idiots, and raised their fists in return.

They would make their way to the Black Hills of South Dakota in no particular hurry, giving the newer riders time to become one with their machines. At the Sturgis Motorcycle Rally, Frank and Nicolai plunge deeper still into the subculture that would be their cover, and then …

But in that glorious moment, those thoughts were far from their minds.

ACKNOWLEDGEMENTS

In writing *Good Shrink/Bad Shrink* I drew upon over forty years of study, research, and practice experience in psychiatry, psychoanalysis, and medical hypnosis.

Estelle Sacknoff Kluft, my wife of nearly fifty years, hails from Fall River, Massachusetts. My brother-in-law and friend Harvey Reback, M.D., and my late sister-in-law, Sylvia Reback, and more recently Harvey and Elaine Reback, often hosted my family in Somerset. My daughter, Jacqueline, lived for many years in Falmouth. Teaching continuing education summer courses for the Department of Psychiatry at Harvard Medical School, under the direction of Larry Lifson, M.D., afforded me many opportunities to explore Cape Cod, Martha's Vineyard, and Nantucket.

Accompanying my wife to Durfee High School reunions introduced me to elements of French-Canadian and Portuguese culture. One of her classmates gave me a "Portuguese" name in jest. That name now belongs to former SEAL Annibal Cabral.

Mary Ellen Sylvia is an amateur genealogist and historian. She generously shared her extensive research into Portuguese culture and genealogy, the persistence of the hidden practice of Portuguese Judaism in the aftermath of the Inquisition, the

Portuguese presence in the maritime industries of Connecticut and Massachusetts, and the history of Stonington, Connecticut. I acknowledge her scholarship and kindness in naming one of the book's heroines, Maryellen Madeiros, in her honor. For the sake of her peace of mind, I must state emphatically that the Portuguese obscenities used in this book, which Peter Souza's grandfather translated into English for Ben Jordan, came from other sources.

Like Peter Sousa, I have stood in fascination watching the whaleboat demonstrations at the Museum of America and the Sea in Mystic Seaport, and will stand there in fascination again.

I am indebted to Jeannie Whitman Perkins, director of customer relations, and David Maynard, of James A. Purdey & Sons Ltd., at Audley House in Mayfair, London. I knew there were several plot-relevant matters regarding firearms about which I was uninformed, and others I feared I had misunderstood, my research notwithstanding. Mr. Maynard clarified these matters in words and helped me understand them more completely by allowing me to actually handle the kind of side-by-side Purdey shotgun Eve Gilchrist uses in this book. He saved me from leaving several inaccuracies uncorrected.

I am grateful to several of the good people at Karnac Books for their consistently constructive and supportive contributions, with special thanks to Mr. Rod Tweedy and Mrs. Kate Pearce along the way. I was especially fortunate to work with Mr. James Darley. His meticulous editorial scrutiny of the manuscript of *Good Shrink/Bad Shrink* and his helpful suggestions were gifts of profound value. In addition, Mr. Darley was kind enough to provide me with much-needed additional education about firearms and aspects of shooting relevant to improving this book. Any remaining errors are mine alone.

Several of the names in this book refer to historical figures. New Orleans surgeon Dabney Ewin pioneered the use of hypnosis to reduce burn damage. His contributions play a crucial role in this book. Dr. Ewin gave me useful feedback on my extension (and perhaps overextension) of his work to containing the damage of chemical burn injuries. George Estabrooks wrote early and openly about military uses of hypnosis. Alan Scheflin and his associates did heroic work in uncovering abuses by mental health professionals conducting studies for covert agencies. The late Lester Luborsky, a preeminent psychotherapy researcher, was a mentor with whose research team I worked for several years. Aaron T. "Tim" Beck, another mentor, is the father of modern cognitive therapy. Otto Kernberg ranks among the greatest of twentieth-century contributors to psychoanalytic thinking. Arthur Blank's work on the unconscious flashback phenomenon is a valuable advance in understanding post-traumatic psychopathology. Martin Orne, Ernest Hilgard, Andre Weitzenhoffer, and Milton Erickson were luminaries in the study of hypnosis. Erickson is widely considered the most brilliant practitioner of clinical hypnosis in the modern era. Henri Ellenberger's *The Discovery of the Unconscious* is a remarkable history of dynamic psychiatry. The names of other psychiatric and psychological figures in this book are apocryphal.

My thanks to all of those mentioned above, and to many others who were helpful and generous, but whose names I have forgotten over the years, or who preferred to remain anonymous. Long-time friends who have read my manuscript insist that the voice of Richard "Dick" O'Connell, my soccer coach at Rutgers Preparatory School, comes through loud and clear in Coaches Fletcher and Buchholz.

I thank as well the many gifted writers whose work I have enjoyed, and who have influenced my writing. In particular, I thank Tess Gerritson and the late Michael Palmer, my teachers in a very productive SEAK course on writing for physicians.

ABOUT THE AUTHOR

Richard P. Kluft practices psychiatry, psychoanalysis, and medical hypnosis in Bala Cynwyd, Pennsylvania. He is clinical professor of psychiatry at Temple University School of Medicine, and also teaches at the Psychoanalytic Center of Philadelphia. His contributions on trauma, hypnosis, and the dissociative disorders have earned many recognitions, including the 2009 Pierre Janet Award for Clinical Excellence from the International Society of Hypnosis. The *American Journal of Clinical Hypnosis* awarded him its Milton Erickson Award for best paper of the year on four occasions. Recent books include *Shelter from the Storm*, a meditation on abreaction, and *How Fievel Stole the Moon—A Tale for Sweet Children and Sour Scholars*, a reflection on the ethics and mores of scholarly discourse.